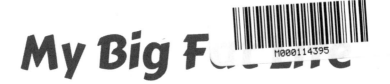

# My Big Fat Life

## *Transformation*

I Defied Mainstream Logic to Lose More than 100 Pounds and Let Go of Yo-Yo Diets Forever!

# Nissa Graun

### From

### *Eating Fat is the New Skinny*

# Dedication

This book is dedicated to all women who have been told to eat far too little and work out way too much to get "healthy." Please know, there is a better way.

# Introduction

For more than 20 years conventional diet wisdom failed me. For two decades I followed all of the rules. Year after year, diet after diet, promise after promise, I failed miserably. I blamed myself. The diet industry blamed me too. There were plenty of fingers pointed swiftly in my direction.

I did not find health and diet freedom until I pointed my longest finger straight into the air to give traditional diets and all of their conventional promises a proper one finger salute.

I am not a doctor. I am a mere former fat girl who dusted the Dorito crumbs from her 2XL sweater, opened a book filled with unconventional ideas and opened her mind to new possibilities. I was on the wrong side of health and endured relentless yo-yo diets for decades. Doctors did not help me. Commercial weight loss programs left me with abysmal results. The media steered me in every direction except the right one.

Since I have no plans to attend medical school, nothing in this book is to be taken as medical advice. When doctors failed me just as I needed them most, I cancelled my appointments and did my own research. I can only suggest you research your own health as well.

I followed the exact opposite advice supplied by the mainstream. I moved less and ate more. I ditched cardboard flavored dinners for juicy steaks topped with butter and dark chocolate desserts. This is what it took to regain my health and fit into a size 6 jeans for the first time in my life. I have never been in better health, nor have I ever felt better in my own body than I do today.

While it is my duty to inform you to follow the advice your doctor provides, as this book progresses my passion for real health will come through. Real health is much different than what the mainstream presents as health. My quest to spread the truth at times will override the information most people are not willing to write about in order to maintain the status quo. Newsflash: maintaining the status quo keeps us fat.

Also, these are my truths. Keep in mind throughout this book that we are all different. Everything that works well for my body may not work as well for your body, but you will never know until you try. You can never try unless the information is provided to you.

I am by far not the first person to lose weight and regain health via unconventional methods. I am definitely not the first person to write a book about it. So why write yet another book about the path to diet freedom and amazing health? Because it is *my* path and there is no other story out there that is exactly the same. Much like snowflakes and fingerprints, everyone's journey to true health is different. My hope is to inspire those reading this who have not yet solidified their path. I also want to connect with so many others who have had a lifetime of struggle and may find solace that they are not alone. While some of my steps may vary from yours, perhaps you can learn something from my successes and even more from my failures.

Besides, this book is not just another fitness expert shaming you into her food choices or his workouts in order to become his or her clone. Let's face it, most of those people have never seen the inside of a Jenny Craig Center. Seriously, do you think any one of the experts you admire ever sucked in his or her gut while holding back tears for a shameful before pose, only to never quite make it to the celebrated after photo? Because I have. More than once. I have been in the trenches. In fact, I have dug myself out of the trenches so many times before that I should have the arm strength to bench press a semi truck by now.

There is also a lot of horrific advice given regarding weight loss and health by people many view as leading health authorities. For more than twenty years I followed most of this advice, only to become sicker and fatter each year. While no one "diet rule" is right for every single person, there is still a whole lotta malarkey out there that should not be told to anyone. It continues to be repeated. It continues to be followed. Many people are doing their best only to become sicker and fatter with each new year of struggle. Then they are blamed for not following health advice correctly, when the truth is the advice was never sound advice in the first place.

I recently read a statistic that less than five percent of people who lose a significant amount of weight will keep the weight off long term. Most people regain the weight they lost, plus additional pounds, within the first year. For more than twenty years I lead the pack in that statistic. Almost every single year I worked hard to lose somewhere between twenty to fifty pounds. Many of those years I was successful at melting away some of the fat.

There are two important notes to make here: 1. I never made it to an official goal weight I had set for myself and 2. I always gained the weight back by the same time the following year. Usually more. Yep, I was the statistic everyone talks about; just another sad, unhealthy, fat statistic.

My ultimate path to health did not begin like most other stories you hear. There was no defining rock bottom moment where I threw my arms up in despair, desperately emptied my pantry of all twinkies and twizzlers, and vowed to conquer my weight once and for all. There was no big declaration because after more than twenty years worth of heartbreaking attempts, I was defeated. I did not believe I was meant to be at a healthy weight and I definitely did not entertain the possibility of ridding myself of years of chronic poor health. At this point in my life, my ultimate goal was to accept my situation as my new normal while taking care of my tiny bundle of joy.

You read that correctly. I was the absolute sickest and fattest version of myself right as I was entering into my new role of motherhood. Topping the scales at more than 245 pounds on a 5'7 frame, I. Was. Fat. As harsh as that may sound coming from a new mother who is supposed to be all namaste while entering the most joyous and anticipated time of her life, it was the truth. Twenty years of diet debacles finally caught up with me and made me officially morbidly obese.

Wow. Morbidly obese. That is hard to see in writing.

Even as a reformed lifetime yo-yo dieter, those are words I actually never thought I would say out loud. At least not about myself. Sure, I was always the chubby girl and at times even the fat friend of my circle, but I was always a mere Weight Watchers stint away from getting back into my single digit jeans. Of course I always kept the comfy size 10's, 12's and 14's handy just in case, but I typically could diet down back into those 8's, at least for a month or two. Everytime I lost the weight, I swore it would be for good. My weight loss victories never lasted long.

When I became pregnant in December 2012, I was actually at the highest weight I would allow for myself before attempting the newest diet craze. The scale hovered around 180 pounds. This seems almost unbelievable since I worked so hard to weigh in a little less than 150 pounds only eight months prior. I know I was smaller because I had to squeeze into my stunning Vera Wang gown. OK, so maybe I make my wedding dress sound a little more glamorous than it was.

While still absolutely gorgeous, it is not one of those designer Vera Wang gowns that someone far snootier than myself would nonchalantly plop down more than ten thousand dollars to wear one time. This girl from the tiny village of Worth, Illinois just didn't have that kind of cash. My dress was from the new David's Bridal Vera Wang Wedding Dress Collection.

That being said, it was still beautiful and absolutely made for me. I know this to be true since the male dress attendant gushed that I was the most beautiful bride he saw in that dress since it arrived at the store a few days prior. I'm sure it had nothing to do with the fact those employees work largely on commission. Nothing at all. He gushed; I whipped out my credit card for the very first dress I tried on. It was love at first sight. Only seeing my newborn son for the first time evoked such strong emotions as seeing myself in a dress drenched in fluffy ivory tulle and embroidered flowers. (Sorry husband, it's just a different kind of love).

That entire tangent was just to say that somehow I gained more than thirty pounds in less than eight months. Again. And this time I could not even hit up my pals Kirstie Alley or Valerie Bertinelli to take it off because I found out I was with child. (I love how dramatic that sounds). I went into my very first pregnancy tipping the scales at my highest weight ever.

I waited a lifetime to become pregnant, although not for the sappy reasons you might assume. Sure I wanted a child to cuddle and nurture and all of that mushy-gushy stuff, but my real daydream of pregnancy was that momma finally got to eat! After more than twenty years of long droughts void of my favorite foods while carefully monitoring calories, followed by brief desperate periods of shoving every nacho chip and cheese fry I could round up into my mouth, followed by even more dieting, more struggle and more pain, I was ready to just eat without restrictions.

My dreams of swimming in endless bags of Cool Ranch Doritos and ordering up daily Big Mac Meals hit a harsh reality when I found out that you actually are supposed to eat an even healthier diet when you are pregnant to ensure you produce a healthy offspring. Roadblock number one. Roadblock number two was my cravings completely changed when I was pregnant. Plain carbohydrates, like spaghetti and toast, were sometimes the only thing I could choke down. Even when I ate the foods that would settle my growing belly, I could never really eat very much. After a just a few bites I was so full that I felt like I just spent three hours at Maggiano's with my overzealous stepdad who tended to order the entire restaurant menu for our small family of eight.

So there I was, a weebly, wobbly pregnant lady who kept growing despite barely managing to eat what I feed my picky toddler over the course of a day now. The carbohydrate rich foods he prefers aren't much different than what I ate either. Not surprisingly, with my pregnant lady I-need-more-carbs-or-I-am-going-to-puke state of being, as well as my waistline expanding far more than it should have with only one baby growing inside, my pregnancy health was not the best. Not only did I pack on more than sixty pounds over the course of the ten month pregnancy, (yes guys, it really is closer to ten months than nine) but I also was diagnosed with gestational diabetes.

When the doctor first called with the news, I didn't really think it was that big of a deal. Then Google came into play. As it turns out, pretty big deal. Like your baby could die big deal. Let me add right here if you are a five month along pregosaurus emotional mess, do not use Google to assess your diagnosis. Follow the directions of your doctor and leave it at that. But only if you have a good doctor who believes in more patient care than just doling out medications for your symptoms, followed up by prescribing additional medications for the new symptoms that arise from the first prescription given. Then find a new doctor and follow his or her advice.

Cut to me being sawed in half with my newborn son being ripped from my womb. With a dozen masked hospital personnel watching over my fully exposed nether regions in an extremely frigid and brightly lit room, I couldn't imagine a more beautiful moment. (Induced births and c-sections are sometimes also a part of gestational diabetes). This was about the same time I had to come to terms with the fact that I somehow reached the poorest health of my life. Not a great way to start my new chapter.

After returning home with this baby who I loved immensely, but had absolutely no idea what to do with, I allowed myself a few months to settle into my new situation. Nobody prepares you for the months of only having a few minutes of sleep each hour because you have to wake to feed the baby. Or perhaps a lack of to sleep due to your refusal to close your eyes, because as soon as you close your eyes you know in your heart that your baby is going to spontaneously die. While he has zero health issues and cannot even roll onto his side yet, you fear he will randomly suffocate if you are unable to analyze his every breath all night long. They now make devices to track this, so I know I am not the only one with an overactive mommy imagination.

No one issues a warning about the dishes and dust that pile up because you cannot leave the couch for hours at a time as your newborn nuzzles his tiny head on your chest. A life with this helpless being who utterly depends on you in order to thrive requires an adjustment period which should be free of typical life stresses of the past. I allowed myself just that before the extra weight started weighing on my mind once again.

During those late night feedings and hours spent snuggling my newborn, I had a lot of time to think. I lived so much of my life in this never ending calorie struggle. I spent so much money on failed diet programs and coaches and personal trainers I never used and tasteless diet foods I could barely choke down, only to be in a far worse position than where I started many years before.

I thought about all of the work I previously put into obtaining my goal body and gasped at how I could possibly maintain such an obsessive lifestyle while having this new baby in my life. I came to the realization that I could not, or at the very least would not, re-enter that diet obsessed world that was my life for more than twenty years. My baby boy deserved all of my obsessive attention on him and him alone. Counting calories and mainstream diet programs no longer deserved my precious energy.

More than anything, I just wanted a normal life. I observed so many people that just eat food. They didn't measure their meals with cups or a clunky kitchen scale. I never saw them stopping to add every bite they just consumed into food apps on their phones. They were not spending five minutes picking out the carb laden noodles in their salads, even though their brains were screaming out for even just one desperate bite. They eat normal food and they go on to wear the same size clothing year after year without much effort. I wanted that life, even if that meant the size of my clothing would now be double what I considered to be a normal size.

That was the life I resigned to after coming to terms with my heaviest weight ever. In the back of my mind I still desperately yearned to take off the weight, but I was far too drained to fight any longer. My days of desperation to rid myself of my muffin top needed to come to an end once and for all. After twenty years of struggle, I succumbed to my plus sized life.

After more than two-thirds of my life spent in the diet game, where I swear to you I was a straight A student, how did morbid obesity become my reality?

# Find Your Optimal

# Health

As you can see by the photo on the cover of this book, I did not bury my head in the sand while hiding my oversized body in clearance specials from the Torrid clothing rack for the rest of my days. I unwillingly lived too much of my life hiding from cameras and tugging tight fitting clothing out of my fat rolls. After a few months of researching the newest and flashiest diet trends, I accidentally came across a free book on Amazon called *Kick Your Fat in the Nuts.* I did not know it at the time, but the direction of my life was about to be forever changed...in the best possible way.

I found out most of the nutrition information I eagerly studied for more than twenty years came from biased studies performed by food companies or even the government we trust to guide us. I decided to throw all conventional diet wisdom away and start from scratch with the new ideas presented to me in this book, as well as other sources I stumbled upon.

It has been more than four years since I started over with these new information sources. Not only did I lose more than 90 pounds after my first pregnancy and another 65 pounds after my second pregnancy, but I regained my health after desperately struggling with everything from daily migraines to constant anxiety, depression, cystic acne and much more for the majority of my life.

All of these improvements came into my life because I went against the grain by no longer consuming "healthy whole grains."

I sit before you today a completely changed person. Never in my life did I believe it would be so easy to maintain a weight loss of more than 100 pounds from my heaviest weight. I never even thought to dream of this healthy, happy and energetic life I finally find myself living after a lifetime of struggle. The older I get, the younger I feel. Many of the strategies I present in this book can truly help you age in reverse.

Nearly one year ago I set out on a mission to guide and help others make the exact changes I did so they can find their own fountain of youth. Many of the articles you will read throughout this book have been published on my website eatingfatisthenewskinny.com. With this book I hope to guide the reader through the articles in order to help piece them together and show how this information can be utilized to transform your life just as I have transformed mine. I will take breaks in between blogs to explain how I applied the information presented for my inspirational weight loss and optimal health gains.

The first blog in the series *Stubborn, Sucky Baby Weight* is the place where anyone new to low-carb, high-fat diets should start. While ketogenic diets are all the rage these days, jumping right into a ketogenic diet can throw many people's bodies into complete shock. This can make for a miserable low-carb, high-fat experience. Sometimes it can even lead to weight gain.

When you begin a low-carb, high-fat lifestyle, these are changes you want to make for life. Give your body and mind time to adjust with the simple steps outlined in the first blog. Once you are ready to step it up, go for it! This book contains several different ways to progress your health as you are ready to do so.

Even if you are not a mom trying to lose stubborn baby weight, do not skip over this article. There is important information outlined in the blog that can help you begin your life transformation on the right track.

# *Stubborn, Sucky Baby Weight*

Pregnancy pounds – they suck. You know what is even suckier than sucky pregnancy pounds? The constant yo-yo dieting pounds already accumulated before the baby was even a tiny twinkle in your eye, but then you added the pregnancy pounds too. And I'm talking over twenty years of yo-yoing up, down, and that big old loop de loop really talented yo-yo magicians can do.

I guess you can say I am no stranger to this whole dieting game. I mean, who among us hasn't tried every diet gimmick known to woman in an attempt to squeeze into jeans you should have thrown in the towel on twenty pounds ago? And if you are in the corner raising your hand because you are a rare specimen that can shove an entire plate of extra cheesy nachos down, followed by a large Coke and not gain an ounce, go somewhere else. Ain't nobody got time for you and your nachos while attempting to read a fat girl blog, in between demanding her toddlers quit jumping on the couch for the fourteenth time.

But I digress. Pregnancy pounds are the worst and pretty much impossible to lose. They continue to compound with each kid and before you know it, you start to wonder if the airline is going to make you purchase an extra seat this year for holiday travel – and I'm not talking about for your kids under two, mmmmkay?

Deep down you know there is nothing you can do about it. You already crawled on hands and knees back to Weight Watchers because Oprah told you that you can eat bread. *BREAD!* Somehow counting all the points in the world just isn't cutting it anymore. Looks like those XXL maternity pants are here to stay.

Been there, done that, never doing it again.

# The "Expert" Advice

So you know all of that advice the experts dole out about having to make diet changes into a lifestyle change? After more than twenty years on the diet roller coaster I finally learned they are absolutely right. It took me multiple rounds of Slimfast, Weight Watchers and Jenny Craig to figure that out. Do you know what other advice the experts dole out that they are also absolutely right about? Pretty much nothing else.

I cannot claim myself an expert in the field of nutrition, but I am a bonafide health geek. I listen to every reliable health podcast out there and read all about the latest health breakthroughs, in between yelling at my toddlers to quit jumping on the couch, again. Always desperate to find something to keep the pounds off, I have always read every article I could find pretty much since I was twelve. The difference is I finally sifted through the expert BS and found the real answers that really work! A feat more than twenty years in the making.

I am unsure why I feel the need to keep pointing out that I was stuck in diet mentality for over twenty years. I will quit beating around that tree of broccoli decomposing in your produce drawer and just spell it out – I am old. I am an older mom of very young kids, but with age comes wisdom…or something.

We're friends, right? I mean, I popped out two kids; I am guessing you popped out at least one since you are still reading this. At the very least, we have all had food babies in our bellies at some time or another. We are probably both sitting on our couches right now contemplating what fabulous dinner we should slave over only to have our toddlers throw it all on the floor. That's a friend in my book! These days, anyway.

Since we are friends, I want to help you. I don't want you to struggle with health or weight issues any longer. And since we are both busy moms, or gestators of food babies, I want to make it easy for you. Let me break it down.

# *Good Health Is Not Hard*

The reason I said none of the advice the experts give is right is that every expert tells you something different. When you are fed up with one expert's advice, you move onto the next; then back to the previous; and then you end up chowing down an entire bag of Cool Ranch Doritos in tears while searching out yet another expert's advice.

This does not lead to health gains; it leads to frustration. Cold, lonely, eat an entire tray of brownies topped with extra fudge frustration. I have good news. Good health is not that complicated. Good health is not found in daily health shakes, protein bars, endless elliptical sessions or the supplement aisle at Walgreens. (Please, please do not buy your supplements at Walgreens. If you'd like, I can pick you up and speed down the 202 while blasting some Brittany and throw your hard earned cash directly out the window. That would at least provide some entertainment while throwing away your money).

Good health is found in the choices you make everyday by choosing to feed yourself and your family real, whole foods. But wait, you didn't think all of that lead up was for that little gem of advice, did you? Of course there is more to the story. Much, much more, but like I said, we are going to keep it simple at first. It has to be simple in order to become your new lifestyle.

To begin your new journey to excellent health, start with baby steps. Throw away every useless piece of advice you learned from the experts. Stop counting calories. Quit looking at fat grams (unless you are looking to add more healthy fats, because healthy fats are key to excellent health). No more logging hours upon hours on the treadmill. Heck, if you are really feeling brave, throw away your scale.

Just sttttaaaaahhhhpppp! Stop the dieting madness and mentality. It's a trap, I swear. Having lost 90 pounds after my first pregnancy and another 65 after my second pregnancy, while finally being able to keep it off and feeling great in the process, I can attest it is a trap. It is a time trap, a money trap, a fat trap. A big scam to keep you overweight and unhealthy and coming back for more.

## 3 Simple Rules

As I said above, there is much more to this health journey, but we all need to start somewhere. If you are sick and tired of feeling sick and tired and fat, there are only three rules beginners should follow. Clear your cluttered mind of everything else you learned about health to this point.

*Rule 1:* Forget what all of the experts tell you about constantly needing food to shove into your face to give you energy and to "stoke" your metabolism. This benefits the food companies and the food companies only. From this point on be sure you are eating only in a 12 hour window. What I mean by this is, if you have your first bite of food at 7 am, then you should not have anything else after 7 pm. Keep a 12 hour eating window most days of the week.

*Rule 2:* I know you don't want to hear this, but it has to be said. Yes, you need to cut back on all of those yummy carbohydrates. Yep, even the "healthy" whole wheat carbohydrates the experts have been touting for decades. Yep, even fruit and fruit juice carbohydrates; especially fruit juice carbohydrates!

It's not all bad news. You get to keep *some* of your beloved carbs. Starting out, your goal should be to eat 25 grams of carbs or less per meal for most of your meals each day. The occasional cheat meal, meh, you can probably get away with it – but I do mean occasional as in a holiday or birthday meal, not occasional as in three times each week meal.

*Rule 3:* Educate yourself. Never stop educating yourself to help you find what works for your body. **Everyone is different and has different needs**. No one diet is going to work for everyone. (Sorry experts cashing in on useless products, ain't gonna happen).

Become a health geek. Listen to the reliable podcasts and read the unsponsored articles. I know there is a ton of information out there, but stick with me and I will point you to the good stuff. Rules 1 and 2 are pretty general and a really great start, but you need to build from there to help you find what is best for you.

That is it. Start with those three rules to get yourself on the path of success today. No more waiting for Monday. The rules are so easy that you can start with your next meal.

Ok, gotta run. My toddlers just went from jumping on the couch to jumping on each other.

# Start With Easy

While at first glance, you may think *Stubborn, Sucky Baby Weight* is meant only for new mothers who have trouble dropping the pregnancy pounds, it really is applicable to anyone who is trying to lose weight with the typical diet dogma, but has had very little success via conventional methods.

After basing our diets on the government provided food pyramid for so long, many of us have developed insulin resistance. If we continue to base our diets on "healthy" whole grains, pastas, cereals and other processed carbohydrates, our waistlines will continue to expand and diseases like Type 2 Diabetes may start to come into play sooner rather than later.

Starting the simple process of lowering your carbohydrate intake and limiting your window of eating each day can go a long way in reversing both the weight gain and possibly even the onset of metabolic diseases like Type 2 Diabetes.

Once again, I am not a doctor. I have never been to medical school and never plan to go. I can tell you before I started the process of lowering my carb level and beginning an intermittent fasting eating schedule, I was on the path to Type 2 Diabetes. My blood sugar levels were already there. The only thing I did not have was an official diagnosis.

I began with the steps outlined in *Stubborn, Sucky Baby Weight.* Soon enough my blood sugars were back in normal ranges in just a few months without medications. Food and time heal. Always take the advice of the doctor you choose...but be very choosy of your doctor.

If you want to stay with only 25 grams of carbs per meals for most meals and 12 hour eating windows for the next few months, do it!

Always do what feels right for your body and do not rush this process.

In my previous yo-yo dieting past I tried low-carb diets many times. I consistently failed at low-carb diets because I always rushed into the hard part (over-restricting carbs and calories) hoping that the weight loss would come more quickly. My body was not ready for the hard part, resulting in failure each time I gave my best effort.

It was not until I came across the book *Kick Your Fat in the Nuts* and the 12 Week Online Fat Loss Course that I realized I would always fail at low-carb diets because my body could not properly digest fat and protein. Once I gave myself time to adjust to eating 25 grams of carbs per meal instead of per day, low-carb diets suddenly became way easier to follow. You must also take into account I was simultaneously following the steps necessary to improve my digestion so my body was able to burn fats and proteins more appropriately.

When you are ready to step up your game, taking steps to improve digestive malfunctions should be next, followed by possibly introducing a ketogenic diet. The difference between the low-carb, high-fat diet detailed above and a ketogenic diet will be thoroughly explained in the next article: *Low-Carb Vs. Ketogenic: The Big Fat Difference.*

# Low-Carb vs. Ketogenic: The Big Fat Difference

I have been eating, breathing and living diet trends for as long as I can remember. I always wanted to reach that mystical diet utopia where I looked good in a bikini and could still throw down my beloved chicken tenders and fries on the regular. I desperately needed to get rid of the maternity bathing suit I was holding onto "just in case" for good. It took far too much time and far too much effort, but better late to the low-carb party than never, I suppose. I finally discovered the piece of the puzzle I was missing all along.

I know if you are reading this, you have likely faced this struggle. Maybe you aren't holding onto your maternity suit because you cannot find a regular swimsuit to hide your fat appropriately. Maybe you refuse to get into a bathing suit at all. I have a three year old, so I don't have that option. The endless whining I would endure would surely drive me mad.

I have good news! My mid-section was finally introduced to the sun this summer for the very first time. For a mom of two who is approaching 40, I wasn't too shabby. I even felt a little confident. Sure, I was only in my backyard swimming with the three year old, but the new neighbors could have peeked over the brick fence at anytime. I assure you, I. Was. Brave.

If you have been following along, many of you know I finally reached my personal health utopia thanks to keto! For anyone who still thinks keto is some sort of supplement sold by MLM companies, read on. I have an entire blog on deck dedicated to the keto newbies of the world.

Now I want you to fully prepare yourself for shock and awe with this next statement I am going to make. ***A ketogenic diet alone was not responsible for the majority of my success.***

The lies! The trickery! Everyone wants their money back!

Wait a minute, this is all free.

Ok, so it's not all that shocking, especially since I have alluded to that, as well as flat out written about that, in several other blogs. Long before I followed a ketogenic diet, I was simply low-carb. Guess what – being simply low-carb is sometimes enough. I lost 90 pounds with being simply low-carb after my first pregnancy. I didn't know what a ketogenic diet was until then. Sometimes simple is all it takes. Well, until I find out it's not quite as simple as I thought.

## My Low-Carb, High-Fat Path

I am fortunate to have had many people reach out to let me know I have inspired them to continue their health journey. Still, I have many others that do not know what in the bologna sandwiches I am talking about. I do not endorse bologna sandwiches and I clearly watch far too much Mickey Mouse Clubhouse.

Here is the basic timeline I used to finally reach my goal weight for the first time after struggling for more than twenty five years:

- **September 2013** – reached highest weight after birth of son.
- **February 2014** – Read Kick Your Fat in the Nuts (and then re-read it a few more times). Began natural supplements to fix digestive issues. Began reducing carbohydrates to less than 25 gram per meal for most meals and snacks. Added more healthy fats to diet. Reduced eating windows to 10-12 hours per day.
- **February 2015** – lost 60 pounds by this point. Digestive supplements and better diet fixed a multitude of health problems that plagued me for decades. Heard about ketogenic diet.

- **March 2015** – began reducing carbohydrates from approximately 100-150 per day to approximately 20-30 per day. Ate even more fat.
- **June 2015** – lost additional 30 pounds by this point. Some days were low-carb, while others were considered ketogenic. Became pregnant with second child.
- **June 2015 – March 2016** – kept processed carbs low, kept healthy fats high, went for walks. Gained approximately 50 pounds during pregnancy. Avoided gestational diabetes.
- **April 2016** – began lowering carbs to ketogenic levels. Resumed frequent walks.
- **August 2016** – sold house and moved across country with two small children. Food free for all!
- **October 2016** – began reducing carbs to ketogenic level.
- **December 2016** – Christmas break in Chicago. Food free for all.
- **January 2017** – resumed low-carb, high-fat, ketogenic diet. Began experimenting with longer periods of intermittent fasting. (Went from daily 16:8 to some weeks with at least 1-2  24 hour fasts per week)
- **April/May 2017** – reached goal weight of 135 pounds. Total weight lost after second pregnancy 65 pounds + 90 pounds from first pregnancy.
- **Determined this stuff works after all.**

As you can see, my diet plan changed from start to finish. I had periods of time where I was simply low-carb, periods of time where I was strictly keto and periods of time where life happened and I ate whatever was shoved in front of my face. Guess what! All of these methods helped me to my goal. Well, not the shoving junk in my face. But it happened and I didn't go all crazy, only to wake up years later with Dorito crumbs falling down my 2X shirt.

I planned for it, I kept it reasonable (which wasn't hard since I fixed my digestion and didn't crave all of the junk of the days of yore) and I picked myself up to get back on my eating plan when I was ready. Sure, eating keto and adding intermittent fasting sped up the results and led to some pretty marvelous health gains including unbelievable energy, but keto wasn't absolutely necessary for me.

As messed up as my hormones were from years of bad diets and too many over the counter medications, I was still fixable and I allowed myself time to heal. For other people, keto is exactly what they need to heal and they cannot afford to veer off course. This is all very individual people.

Since it is individual, I want to explain the differences between low-carb and ketogenic, and what makes each lifestyle work.

## *Low-Carb Diets*

When I began to eat low-carb, which involved cutting my carbs to less than 25 grams per meal, this caused a less severe insulin spike than previous meals of say, spaghetti with meat sauce, which probably has around 50-100 grams of carbs just for the spaghetti and sauce. The spaghetti package says only 42 grams, but who measures out only one cup of spaghetti noodles? And then you add in the garlic bread, maybe a fruit popsicle after dinner. Holy insulin spike Batman!

***When your insulin is hard at work trying to recover from this huge spike, your body is not able to burn fat. Not only is your body not burning fat, it is now storing excess fat.*** So when you take that spaghetti and meat sauce – let's say 75 grams of carbs + garlic bread 25 grams of carbs + fruit popsicle 13 grams of carbs, oh and wait, let's not forget about that Coke you had with dinner too + 40 grams of carbs. That is a 163 grams of carbs spike your body now has to recover from. Well, that's *IF* it ever recovered from the carbs you had at 3 pm because you were so hungry that you would have eaten cookies off the ground if that was your only option. Thank goodness for the vending machine!

When your insulin is spiking up and down ALL DAY LONG because you have to eat ALL DAY LONG because the processed carbohydrates you are consuming make you ravenous ALL DAY LONG, guess what your body never has a chance to do. Burn fat.

So about that diet you keep saying you are on… If you are eating carbs all day, not gonna happen; so quit talking about it already. You are wasting time talking when your internal clock says it's time to find more junk to shove into your pie-hole.

If you want to make that spaghetti and meat sauce meal work on a low-carb diet, let's make a few changes. How about we eat only half of a portion of noodles starting out. Soon enough you can wean them all together, but for now, just eat half. And how about you add some green peppers, onions, zucchini and fat, maybe butter or olive oil, to that low sugar sauce to help fill you up and give your body the nutrition it needs. Get rid of the garlic bread and popsicle. Just because it says it is fruit does not mean it is good for you. Do we even need to talk about the Coke? Liquid sugar in any form is the fastest way to spike your insulin. (Here's looking at you "healthy" orange juice).

Hey you! Yeah you, trying to sneak in that Diet Coke. Uh, uh. Let's stop that right now. Who do you typically see drinking diet sodas? Overweight people. Do you know why that is? Diet soda can also cause insulin spikes, which causes weight gain. And you people with the diet soda didn't even get sugar out of the deal. (Who am I fooling here. It is diet pop. I'm a midwestern girl).

So now that we have taken our meal from over 160 carbs down to only 25 carbs, and we also removed the artificial sweeteners, our body's insulin spike isn't quite so drastic. The body can recover more quickly and can now spend time burning the fat on your body instead of adding more fat to your body. This is called eating for your hormones. **Insulin is the fat storing hormone.** When you eat in a way to bring insulin down, you do not store the fat. Eating 25 grams of carbs or less per meal is one way to bring insulin down. So long calorie counting, I never liked you anyway!

If you eat 25 grams of carbs or less at most meals during the week, your hormones will begin to heal and the weight will start to come off your body accordingly. Be sure to add plenty of healthy fats and proteins to your meals to make you satiated longer.

Every single time you put food in your face, your insulin spikes. Every time your insulin spikes, you are storing fat. If your meals keep you satiated longer, then you can make it to your next meal without a snack. If you are only eating three times per day instead of six times per day, your insulin is spiking only half as many times. (see, even us creative folk can do math). The longer amount of time you give your insulin to rest, **the more opportunity your body has to spend energy burning fat in place of storing fat.**

This low carb thing sounds pretty easy, eh? Sure, at first you might miss all of the sugar a little bit. Who am I kidding? You are probably going to want to rip your spouse's head off due to the sugar withdrawal from your lifelong sugar addiction. If you ever want to heal and get to a healthier place, it's kind of what needs to happen. Kicking the sugar addiction, not ripping your spouse's head off. Once again, fixing the way your body digests food can help here. You can do this the easy way or the hard way. Your choice.

## *KETOGENIC DIETS*

Now we get to keto. Keto is a low-carb diet, but supercharged. Do you know what you get with a supercharged diet? Supercharged results! You are still eating for your hormones, but now you are lowering your insulin level even further! If you get into ketosis correctly and stay there for a while, your hormones begin to heal and you can improve many diseases of civilization, including type 2 diabetes, PCOS, metabolic syndrome, IBS, foggy brain and so much more. I was on the verge of type 2 diabetes. Can you guess how I changed that health sentence. Keto, of course!

With keto you want to lower your carbs all the way down from 100-150 per day to only around 20 per day. Why would you do such a thing? What about the vegetables? What did all the fruits ever do to you, you must be asking. No, I don't hate all the fruits, but they are called nature's candy for a reason. Do you know any reasonable person who goes on a diet and expects to have results eating a bunch of candy? And vegetables, definitely still eat those

– just eat the vegetables lower in carbs and add butter. Lots of glorious, delicious, melted butter! After all, you won't be getting any of the necessary fat soluble vitamins from those vegetables without adding fat.

With keto, you are lowering your carbohydrate intake and replacing it with fat. Like, a lot of fat. And some protein, but not too much. You want to eat 75-85% of your calories from healthy fats. This eventually forces your body to burn fat as fuel instead of glucose, which the majority of people burn. As a glucose burner, your body requires frequent energy boosts in the form of more food all day long. Glucose just isn't an efficient fuel if you have any kind of life and have things to do. Or if you want to burn your stored fat. Glucose sucks as a fuel for burning stored fat.

As a fat burner, you can go for days without additional fuel. Seriously, I have tried it and I felt amazing. It's called intermittent fasting while being fat adapted. Once you are fat adapted, your body breaks through the glucose barrier that needs constant refueling, and starts to burn the fat on your body. Once you are fat adapted, it becomes easy to strategically skip meals because you are finally using the energy up from that Big Mac you had back in 2012. (Thankfully 2012 was the last time I had a Big Mac).

I get many messages from new ketoers telling me they are in ketosis because the pee sticks turned purple. These same people tell me they are on a strict ketogenic diet of less than 100 grams of fat and under 1200 calories. Dear new ketoer, I call that lunch!

I am sorry to be the bearer of bad news, but you are most likely not in ketosis and eating less than 1200 calories per day is no way to heal your hormones. Your body can barely make it out of bed on 1200 calories per day, little lone have the extra energy to heal itself.  There are some days and some people when 1200 calories *might* be enough. The point is, you need to listen to your body – not an app on your phone telling you how many calories you have left for the day. And those purple pee sticks – sorry to tell you, you are most likely dehydrated.

If you are not already on a ketogenic diet, start with low-carb. You can get plenty healthy with a low-carb diet. When you are ready for the amazing benefits of a ketogenic diet, it will actually be easier to make the switch since you are already eating around 100 carbs per day instead of the standard 300+ that most people on a standard diet consume.

## *Low-Carb Vs. Keto*

Some reasons you may want to stay low carb are:

1. **You are not fully committed to a ketogenic diet.** With a keto diet, there is no cheating on the weekends. If you want to get and stay in ketosis, especially at the beginning, it takes work and commitment. Not everybody is ready for that.
2. **Your body is not able to process fats very well yet.** If you feel bloated, gassy, nauseous, have frequent acne, or itchy skin, these are all signs that your body is not digesting the additional fat very well. You may need extra time to ramp up your fat to get anywhere near a ketogenic level. Also, taking Beet Flow or a coffee enema can help speed this process along. (Yes, I said coffee enema. Please seek a professional, because it's not simply streaming coffee into your butt. Well, maybe it is. I was good with the Beet Flow; never needed the enema) Click here for an almost free four week digestion course to learn how these supplements can help you digest fat better.
3. **You are happy with your results from a low-carb diet.** Not everyone wants to be the same size as they were in high school. Some people actually just want healthier insides. Having healthier insides is an awesome goal. Lowering your carbs to under 25 grams per meal can get you here without the extra commitment.

Reasons to start low-carb, then switch to a ketogenic diet:

**1 . You are suffering from any of the diseases of civilization mentioned above.** To eat a ketogenic diet is to heal your hormones. To heal your hormones is to improve your disease.

Real, high quality food will work way better than anything your doctor could ever prescribe. If you are looking for a quick fix, see your doctor. If you are looking for lasting results, change your diet. (NEVER come off your prescribed medications without consulting your doctor).

**2. You want the most energy you have ever felt in your life!** When you adopt a ketogenic lifestyle, your body has almost unlimited fat to use as fuel. You are not constantly experiencing the sugar spikes and crashes of they typical standard American diet. This leads to energy that lasts all day long, without the constant need to refuel.

**3. You want life to be easy without constant food noise.** We have all experienced daydreaming about what you are going to eat for dinner about twenty minutes after we just consumed lunch. When you consume a ketogenic diet, your mind isn't constantly thinking about food. You feel satisfied and can spend your energy on more important tasks. Your brain fog clears and you can accomplish so much more in a day. Throw some intermittent fasting into the mix and look out world, mama's taking over! But that's another blog, another day.

There you have it – the piece of the puzzle I was missing for so long! Low-carb diets and ketogenic diets are both excellent diets for bringing insulin levels down, which helps us burn fat. They just do it at different levels. Choose the results you want, cut back on the junky carbohydrates and eat some coconut oil already!

# Just Eat The

# Coconut Oil

Now that you understand the differences between low-carb, high-fat and a ketogenic diet, you can make the choice of where you want to fall on a daily basis. Or not. You can honestly have a lot of success with just low-carb, high-fat, or with just a ketogenic diet or by mixing and matching the diets according to your life.

Keep in mind falling in and out of ketosis at the beginning can be a difficult transition. If you choose a stricter ketogenic approach, give yourself time before you bounce back and forth. (Typically at least 3-6 months). No one wants to keep entering the keto flu phase every few days. Once you commit to a ketogenic diet, really commit. Once you have been ketogenic for some time, then you will have the ability to be more flexible and have some days that are higher in carbs than others.

I personally followed a low-carb, high-fat diet for at least the first year. I had a lot of success that year. Not only did I drop around 90 pounds, but I was also able to lower my fasting blood sugars from daily averages of 130-140 (diabetic ranges) to normal ranges of 80-90. That's a huge health transformation! And I still was still able to eat some of the carbs my body craved.

After following this way of eating for more than four years, my body enjoys metabolic flexibility. What that means is some days I abide by a strict ketogenic diet where I eat a lot of fat and consume no more than 50 carbohydrates in a day, while other days I get to have a cheat meal of my choice with very little consequence. I cannot say this has always been the case as I had to work hard to get there, but now I reap the benefits of my hard work. Keep working at it and you can enjoy that lifestyle too!

If you are reading through all of this information and your head is absolutely spinning, I got you covered! Knowing that not everyone is quite the health nerd that I am, I created a full six week course that walks you through all of these steps: _Coach Me Course: Escape Diet Mentality and End Yo-Yo Diets Forever._ I have much more information to share with you as this book proceeds, but we are just scratching the surface. If losing a large amount of weight and staying in a healthy range was as simple as saying, "Eat this, don't eat that," we would all have perfect bodies by now!

On to the next article. _Let's Get This Keto Party Started_ is for those of you who are ready for that next step. This is a blog filled with tips I learned over my course of utilizing a ketogenic diet for both the weight loss and health benefits.

If you are not ready for a full-on ketogenic diet, stick with low-carb, high-fat. There is no need to rush the rest of your life. If keto is meant for you, eventually you will make it to a point where you are ready to take the plunge. While a ketogenic diet is a commitment, once you have been low-carb, high-fat for a while, it is a much easier commitment to make.

# Let's Get This Keto Party Started

Keto. Like it or not, keto is a four letter word. See k-e-t-o. Now that we had our morning math, we can move along. Like most four letter words, you can use the term keto when you are ecstatic as f#+& or when you are as angry as $&!+. Some people absolutely love keto and all of the awesome health benefits it provides. Others speak of it as yet another demon fad diet that is sure to end this new civilization that is drowning itself in coconut oil. Those people, I can assure you, either want to keep you sick in order to keep their pockets full, or they tried keto and did it wrong.

Keto is a wonderful way of life where you load up on healthy fats and have more energy than you have ever had in your entire life, while dropping pounds you thought were permanently wedged onto your butt violently by the force of a Mack truck. More importantly, with keto you eat real food.

Unfortunately most of us have never eaten a real food based diet before. Poor June Cleaver is rolling over in her grave to fix you some pot roast and green beans with extra butter and salt. (June Cleaver is dead, right? I didn't just kill her off for the sake of keto, did I?)

While I am not of a fan of the keto fascists of the world telling everyone exactly how they should keto, if you are still eating mostly processed, fast, cheap and easy foods, you are doing it wrong. Mama always said you are what you eat. Please don't be cheap and easy. Let's save that for whoever is pulling rank in Tiger Woods' bed these days.

Sure, you can lose plenty of weight pulling into McDonald's every night, ordering a Mc-something or other and whipping off the bun in a furious keto rage. Many do this, many lose weight, many have well preserved insides from all of the additives in their food. But the keto lifestyle, as I see it, is a lifestyle of optimal health. Just a tidbit of information: optimal health does not come with a side of fries that you plan to lick the salt off of before you toss them into the trash. Come on, have you done this? People don't really do this, right?

## The A-B-C's of K-E-T-O

Let me backup for just a second. Many of you reading this already know the basics of a ketogenic diet. Believe it or not, there are those reading this right now that have no idea what keto is. They do exist! This is the part where I explain keto coated in all of it's saturated fat glory. (Yes I eat saturated fat all day long. Yes I am the healthiest I have ever been).

A well formulated ketogenic diet typically consists of a macronutrient breakdown that amounts to something around 75-85% healthy fats, 10-20% protein and less than 5% carbs. I know what you are thinking. Wholly guacamole, did she just say only 5% carbohydrates? What kind of animals live like that? We have all heard the "experts" recommend a carb based diet for years! Blasphemy, you say!

Umm, have you seen the health of our nation lately? Seems to me the experts are only experts in making us all sick, unhealthy shells of our former vibrant selves. Let's all just quit listening to the experts long enough to experiment with our own health, instead of being lab rats for the experts. Dramatic? Yes! True? Yes!

## My Keto Story:

Before I get to all the good stuff on how to start a ketogenic diet of your very own, let me regale you with the first time I heard about keto and had to rush to try it for myself the very next day! And scene:

My first son just turned 18 months. It was an exciting time for our little family of three since he just started walking the week prior. When I heard about keto on my favorite health podcast, it sounded like the exact, perfect diet I needed in my life at that very moment. I already spent the previous year or so working on my digestion and watching my body slowly shed the layer of fat that once cuddled my first born. In the podcast, the hosts talked about how quickly and easily your body can shed unwanted fluff with a ketogenic diet. Summer was right around the corner and mama wanted out of her maternity bathing suit! I decided to try keto the very next…come on, say it with me now – I started on Monday!

We *ALL* know about Monday diets. Hurry up and shove as much junk into your face as you can until Monday rolls around, then be as strict as you possibly can be. Well, at least until Tuesday, when you've surely lost ten pounds from all of your hard work on Monday!

The only thing worse than a Monday diet is a stupid New Year's Day diet. I mean, really? Why start your brand new you after a night of chugging bubbly and staying out until 4 am to run around the tundra half naked while banging on pots and pans, screaming, "Happy New Year!"? Don't even get me started on all of the alcohol sweat I have had to endure at the gym in order for people to keep their New Year's resolution. Nothing says health like puking out the gin after a good run!

*Tangents. Everywhere I look I see tangents!*

Ok, so my son was 18 months, he just started walking, the day was Monday and my husband was headed off for another week long business trip. I was determined to start my ketogenic diet, but I really had no clue what to eat for breakfast, little lone the rest of my life.

My son woke up a little fussy that day and needed to be held a lot that morning, so I grabbed for something simple – sunflower seeds and a few pieces of dark chocolate. I settled onto my couch, son in one arm and a decent first keto meal in the other. As I reached for my first bite of delicious 88% dark chocolate, I felt a jerk on my other arm, followed by projectile vomit spewing from my sweet baby.

*Projectile vomit. Everywhere I look I see projectile vomit!*

This was the first time my little angel ever had a real sickness in his whole life, and I had to figure it out all on my own because my husband was traveling. Of course my husband was traveling. My son, who had been walking around the house with his hands in the air like he just didn't care for an entire week, suddenly had to be held all day long and carried everywhere. I dreaded leaving my poor baby on the floor for even just a few minutes to use the bathroom. He looked like such a sad, wounded bird. Breaks a mother's heart, it does. And for those of you who are not parents, please know times when your kids are sick are among the most stressful times around.

Who has time to fry up bacon and eggs when you have to tote a projectile vomiting toddler with you everywhere? I did not know exactly what foods constituted keto foods yet, but I am sure any breakfast fried up with a side of toddler vomit was definitely not keto. Can you see me asking on the keto boards if toddler vomit is keto? That would not go over well with the keto fascists.

It is hard to say for sure, but I am pretty confident I ate sunflower seeds and dark chocolate for almost every meal that first week. Not only was I determined to stick with my new ketogenic diet, but by day four I felt like I was hit by a train. Body aches, oh how my body ached. Migraines. I felt hot, I felt cold. Basically I felt like death. And I still had this projectile vomiting buddy attached to my hip every waking hour of the day.

Somehow I stuck with the keto diet for the long haul; or just another few months until I became pregnant with my second child. With my first go around with the keto diet, I did what many people do on a keto diet – I kept my carbs low and then ate stuff with fat in it.

Did I ever reach ketosis in those few months of my first go around? Mmmmm, I dunno. I never tested. The pee strips were purple, but that's about as scientific as I got. There were times when I felt more energy than I had ever felt in my life. I actually felt the urge to clean my house during toddler naps, rather than put my feet up and catch up on the housewives. Anyone who knows me knows I love me some Bravo. My first son was saying Andy Cohen's name long before he acknowledged his daddy. But I actually had so much energy that I couldn't sit still long enough to make it through another argument about who Ramona said hello to first.

Then came my second pregnancy and a strong aversion to meat. So long ketones, I'll miss you. I promise to still write to you from time to time.

After my second pregnancy, I was determined to get back to a ketogenic diet. I had an entire new layer of fat to de-fluff and this time I wanted out of my maternity clothes before people started asking when my baby's Irish twin was due. This time around there was much more information out there, so I decided to make my new keto diet much more official. No more meals of sunflower seeds and dark chocolate for this girl!

## How to Thrive with Keto:

Now that I am a seasoned ketonian, below are some of the things I learned that may be helpful to a beginner. I do not go into all of the basics of a keto diet since there are countless articles and books on this, but here are some tips I had to figure out that might help you:

1.   **Keep your fats high:**   Like even way higher than you think is high. You don't want to go overboard and eat a stick of butter with every meal, but know only adding a teaspoon of mayo over a dry chicken breast is only going to make you hungry and miserable. If you want be hungry and miserable, why even keto? Go measure a dry piece of broccoli or something.

2.  **Change Your Mindset:**  If you are new to keto, but not the dieting world, change your mindset. Quit working out hours upon hours each day. Stop measuring every calorie you put into your mouth. I lost more than 65 pounds after my second baby easy peasy by going for walks every now and then and making sure I was keeping my carbs low. Other than that, no stressful workouts and no calorie obsession. This reset both my mind and my body to feel great while eating the most food I have ever eaten in my life. Not only the most food, but the most delicious food. I swear, I lick the bowl every time I cook. And I can…because I don't count calories!

3.  **Listen to your body:**  Your body truly knows what it wants. If you are hungry, eat some fat. If you feel like you need protein, eat that too. If you really want to eat the entire bag of BBQ chips washed down with a Coke, STOP! You have gone too far! If you are still dealing with these kinds of cravings after being on keto for a few weeks…

4.  **Fix your digestion:**  This was actually my first step and a step I would honestly recommend to anyone before they start any diet, but I get it. Supplements are expensive; fixing digestion takes work; no one wants to take lots of pills. Been there, I totally get it.

Fixing my digestion cleared up so many health problems and I do not believe I ever would have stuck to a low-carbohydrate, high-fat diet without this step. Trust me, I have been trying since the early 2000's. I finally did the work I needed to because taking natural health supplements costs way less now than pretty much even one day in the hospital waiting for my double bypass surgery when I am only forty-something years old. All of the high quality coconut oil in the world means nothing if your body cannot digest it. (To learn more about correcting your digestion, take the almost free four week digestion course found here.)

5.  **Keep your pH levels in check:**  Something else along the lines of working on your digestion is keeping your pH levels in check. This was something I had to learn the hard way. Every single time I did a low-carb diet, I was always getting colds. No, I

do not mean <u>keto flu</u>. I was continually getting sick when I was eating the healthiest I ever had. Before I finished asking myself what was the point, I found an article about pH levels on a keto diet.

Sometimes with a ketogenic diet your saliva pH can drop way too low, and boom! Runny noses and sore throats for days. The article suggested raising your pH by drinking lemon juice or apple cider vinegar. Neither tastes great on their own, so I make a tea with 1 tablespoon apple cider vinegar, 1 tablespoon lemon juice and ½ teaspoon of salt in hot water. It does not taste great the first few times you drink it, but I like it a whole lot better than going through a box of tissues every day for a week.

6.  **Keto Flu:**  Before you even start keto, stock up on avocados, magnesium and a high quality celtic sea or pink himalayan salt. You know the constant bathroom breaks you are taking after dropping a significant amount of carbs from your diet? I have good news. You are not pregnant!!! You are losing electrolytes like crazy, so have them ready to consume on day one.

If you *DO* want to get pregnant, keto helps that as well. Let me go all Oprah for a second – YOU GET A KETO BABY! And YOU GET A KETO BABY! I got my keto baby at the advanced maternal age of 36. Thankfully he was planned. And don't try to tell me age 36 isn't advanced. I saw it on the doctor's paperwork with my own geriatric eyes!

7.  **Quit obsessing about macros:**  I swear, if I see the word macros one.more.time, well, there isn't really anything I am going to do, but just know it makes me mad. Ketones make me feel so happy, so quit ruining that for me! One of the best parts about a ketogenic diet is you do not have to obsess so much about the macros.

Sure, you cannot go hog wild and eat an entire hog, but don't we all understand that already? Let's all put the macro calculators down and start listening to our bodies a little bit more. Some days you need a little bit more protein than others. Some days you are going to eat all the fat, while others you might not want to eat at all. The world is your oyster, but only if oysters are keto. I never checked into that.

My general rule for starting out is to keep your carbs right around 20 (total, not net – net is for cheaters and nobody likes cheaters. Sorry, they just don't) and keep your fats high. Eat fat until you no longer feel hungry, but not until you are stuffed. At the beginning, the protein will just kind of fall into place. You may need to tweak it down the road if you stall or lose your ketones, but just keep it reasonable and there is no reason to obsess.

Some call this method lazy keto. I call it living life.

**8.    Too Many Keto Cooks Whipping Up Advice:**   As with anything that becomes popular, there are far too many keto cooks in the kitchen. One keto group tells you to strictly limit your fat so you only burn your body fat (this friends, will never work); while another keto group tells you to only eat a strict caloric keto diet below 1200 calories (that friends, will never work). A different group tells you that you need boot camp workouts until your legs fall off (Come on? Don't you like having legs?); while a different group will tell you with keto you can lose weight with a simple fasted walk every now and then (THIS ONE! This one is absolutely true! Follow the group that tells you this). The Eating Fat is the New Skinny Support Group is that group!

My point is, too many keto cooks in the kitchen is just confusing everybody and no one is getting it right and everyone is failing miserably. Ok, not everyone. I have had pretty good success, but I do not trust every Tom, Dick and Jimmy in the keto groups. If we are talking Jimmy Moore, I trust that Jimmy.

Quit asking random keto groups questions hoping to get the answer you want to hear. No, you cannot eat a triple hot fudge sundae on Monday and get back into ketosis by Tuesday. How do you even know the experience level of these people that really just want a friend, so they throw out random answers? You are risking an incorrect answer that will throw you into the keto death spiral and return you to sipping Slim Fast. (Is Slim Fast still a thing? Maybe they will jump on the bandwagon and make keto Slim Fast. Please don't buy that). Find the smart people who have had success. Ask those people. I am probably one of those people. Try me.

9. **Keto is a lifestyle, not a diet:**   We have all heard this, yes? If you are just looking to lose a few pounds and then return to your former high processed food life, don't bother. It doesn't even make sense to do that. Getting into ketosis isn't always the easiest process and sometimes not the most fun. (I mean, unless you are doing it with a coach, ahem).

Be into keto for the positive health benefits keto brings – amazing energy, amazing inner healing, amazing weight loss and amazing health gains. In order to make keto your new lifestyle, you need to make it convenient to your life. Prepare to keto. You have to have keto foods in your fridge ready to eat so you are not reaching for the junky stuff. This is not a diet you can cheat on willy nilly. It just doesn't work that way, so be prepared and make it fit your lifestyle or else prepare for a miserable keto experience.

10. **Don't Wing It:**   Do not just wake up one day and decide today is the day you keto and you are going to push through the keto aches and pains no matter what. If you are not already well into your keto diet, break in slowly. There is no reason to rush the rest of your life.

Start by reducing your carbs to a manageable level at first so your body has time to adjust to its new fuel of fat. Start reducing your eating window to 12 hours per day. This actually used to be normal. Today some view it as insane to go 12 whole hours without a lick of food.

Do we need to discuss June Cleaver again? Man, that seems like so long ago when we talked about her. Did anyone google if she is still alive?  If you are still trying to figure out what I mean by reducing your carbs, check out my beginner's blog. I swear it is not the length of this book, er, blog.

**11.    Keep Keto Simple:**   If you are just beginning keto, everybody has got to chill on making replacements for our old favorite junk foods. The more exotic ingredients you bring into your keto diet, the more slippery that slope becomes to just fall back into your old habits. Until you really have this keto thing down, maybe just eat some bacon. Eggs are good. Have you tried eggs lately? Veggies, butter, red meat, pork, salad greens, olive oil, avocados; I can go on and on and on. Keto is all about the real foods! Real foods are yummy. Eat real foods for a while. Use herbs and seasonings. Find some recipes for keto sauces made from fats like heavy whipping cream, pesto and butter.

Sure, I eat fat bombs some days as meals, but I grew into that. I started with the real food, and once I knew what it felt like to be in ketosis, I then began experimenting with all of the keto goodies. I instinctually knew if there was a sweetener or ingredient that was spiking my insulin because I first knew how amazing I felt before I ate the ingredient, and how crappy I felt after. But you need to know this for yourself for awhile before you can make that determination.

It all goes back to listening to your body – but you cannot listen to a body that you never gave a chance to heal because you *HAD* to have a bread replacement or bust. If you feel this way, go back to the part where I talk about digestion. Once you improve your digestion, bread starts to taste like cardboard. (Former bread addict here; don't touch the stuff now).

**12.    Tune Out The Keto Naysayers:**   The very last thing I want to say to all of my keto beginner friends is quit worrying about what other people think about your new diet. Don't waste time arguing with them about how you are going to go into immediate cardiac arrest if you go anywhere near that juicy steak with melted garlic butter.

Sorry vegans, that's mostly you. There aren't vegans here, are there? My husband has this "dad joke" he loves to tell, "Want to know how to tell if somebody is a vegan? Just wait five minutes, they will tell you!"

Now that we all had a good laugh at Moby's expense, why raise your stress levels arguing on the keto boards over the minutia on how to keto correctly? That is *NOT* how to keto correctly. **Stress = Cortisol Spike = Weight Gain**.

How about you keep doing you and let the results speak for themselves. I know people that gasp in horror when I tell them I just downed 75 grams of saturated fat for lunch. These same people are on five different medications and are at least fifty pounds overweight. Me? I take my natural digestive supplements and some vitamin C. I am definitely the healthiest I have ever been. Don't argue with these people. Let them live their medicated lives. You live your coconut oil truth.

So that, all of that up there, is some of the things I wish I knew when I first started my keto. I know you already forgot half the stuff I said, so go back and read it again when you have another hour to kill. Maybe take notes this time so you don't have to keep wondering about June Cleaver. And if you have no idea who June Cleaver is, don't tell me. It is my birthday this week; I don't need another excuse to feel old. I still remember the days when I was good at making people feel old!

PS, let's all thank June Cleaver because she totally inspired this article.

# Before You Keto...

I got so excited to explain the differences between low-carb, high-fat and keto that we skipped over some of the most important information everyone should apply to their lives for easier weight loss and better health - DIGESTION!

You have already heard me mention digestion a bunch of times throughout the previous blogs, but I haven't taken the opportunity to really explain what I mean. Digestion is way more than just eating and then pooping. That is just the tip of the massive iceberg with how important digesting your food properly is to your health and weight loss goals.

Take this next blog seriously. This was the step I was missing for more than 20 years. Guess what happened to me for those 20 years - a whole lotta yo-yo diets and extremely poor health. Had I known the steps for improving my digestion then and had I realized just how much taking those steps would have changed my life, I would have done whatever TC Hale told me to do...no questions asked!

Improving digestive malfunctions is the number one thing you can do to change your life and health forever...but no one talks about it. Well, I am talking about it now! Pay close attention. This is important.

If you haven't taken the <u>Digestion Course</u> yet, do it! The course costs 50 cents and it can change your life forever. Not many people are teaching this life transforming information. Be glad you stumbled upon this book.

# Digestion: More Than A Four Letter Word

When most people think of digestion, they likely think of eating food and then eliminating that food. Simple as a four letter word: poop. (There are many other four letter words for this, but I will do my best to keep this post clean). For those of you that don't know, there is way more to digestion than these two daily occurrences. If you want to learn the ins and outs of how digestion works, I suggest you pick up the book *Kick Your Fat in the Nuts* or check out this four week digestion course. In the meantime, I will do my best to break it down in much simpler terms so you can understand why it is so important for your health and weight loss goals.

There are many good reasons I constantly reference digesting foods properly in almost everything I write. Most health issues people have today, including weight gain and too many others to list, have to do with the way you digest different nutrients. I learned this first hand when I finally took the steps to improve the way I digest foods. I set out with intentions of dropping weight that was not budging with any other method, but I actually improved many health problems that afflicted me for decades.

These ailments include, but are not limited to decades filled with:

- Chronic heartburn
- Cystic acne
- Frequent migraines and headaches
- Constipation
- Diarrhea
- Gas pains
- Constant junk food cravings
- Frequent sinus infections
- Constant drippy nose
- Itchy skin
- Insomnia

- Nausea, especially when eating heavier foods like red meat
- Constant anxiety
- Depression
- Hypoglycemia
- Diabetic range blood sugars
- Chronic ankle, foot and back pain
- Panic attacks

Yes one person can still be alive even after experiencing all of these symptoms - yes, even when many of these symptoms are all experienced in the same day! . Having a body as temperamental as Chicago's weather is not a pleasant existence. This list of ailments does not even touch on my yo-yoing weight, which fluctuated between the same 20-50 pounds for more than twenty years. When you are rolling your eyes because I mention digestion yet again, just know that I have so many reasons to be thankful I finally took the steps to get my digestion back in working order.

## *I Eat, I Poop, Therefore I Am...*

Are you considering skipping this section because you think you do not have any digestive issues? You eat, you poop; you live to eat and poop another day. I too thought my digestion was fine. I too thought digestion issues were only for my grandparents and all they needed to improve their digestion was eat some Activia. Wrong, I was. So wrong I was.

If you have any of the symptoms listed above or have struggled with your weight, I came here to let you know your digestion needs improvement. Guess what else! *That full list is made up of the health problems I improved.* There are tons of other ailments I did not mention because I never had to face those health problems. Many of the health ailments you deal with daily occur because **your** body is not breaking down food properly.

Think of it like this: if you do not eat, you die. If you eat just enough you live, but you do not flourish. When you start eating the amount and kinds of nutrients your body needs to thrive, you live at your most optimal level.

If lifestyle choices over many years have taken their toll on you, you may be eating enough nutrients to thrive, but instead you feel like a broke down Ford Probe. (My first car was a neon blue Ford Probe - it broke down all of the time, so I feel your pain). The nutrients you consume are not being broken down correctly in order to make it to your cells where you need them in order to operate at your most optimal level.

If your body is not properly breaking down the food you eat, guess what happens to it. Just like when you throw meat into a garbage can, it will rot and ferment until it is no longer recognizable as meat. It is now something toxic that will sit in the garbage can until your neighborhood garbage man comes to collect it. ( Put another way, you will get fat and you will probably have stinky breath and your only friends may be on Facebook because no one wants to smell your stinky breath).

You are not so lucky, especially if you have still stinky breath no matter how many times you rinse your mouth. Much like with the garbage can, if a person is unable to breakdown her food, the food rots and ferments in her stomach. Some of that food will eventually be eliminated, however, some of that food is going to be stored as toxins right in her fat cells. These toxins can eventually be eliminated when the coast is clear, but if she keeps consuming more foods that her body is no longer capable of breaking down, the coast is never clear and the toxins keep getting shoved into fat cells. The fat rolls start to multiply. I am not only talking about your everyday run of the mill junk food; even healthy, organic choices can be toxic to your body if you no longer have the enzymes to break them down correctly.

## *Dear Digestion, Why Can't We Be Friends?*

A few things that cause your body to stop digesting foods correctly include poor nutrition choices, such as processed or fast food, years of yo-yo dieting, medications and aging. Some people will never take the steps to improve digestion and will continue to live with the consequences of having rotting and fermenting food in their bodies. Gas pains, bloating, heartburn and no longer being able to eat some of your favorite foods become the norm. Some people's digestion is so screwed up by the time they are older, they actually resort to eating baby food or survive mostly on nutritional shakes since that food is already broken down. Yes, many of our older friends are buying up the Gerber, and it is not for their grandchildren.

So what can you do to abstain from resorting to strained peas and carrots in your golden years? You need to help your body breakdown the food you consume into usable nutrients. Every person is different, just as every person's digestive strength is different. There are a lucky few who can fix the way their body digests foods just by making better food choices. They can eat less processed carbohydrates, less chemically laden foods and less processed meats. These lucky people instead can opt for grass-fed, hormone free, organic meats, organic fruits and vegetables, and healthy fats like real butter and avocados. That is always the best place to start. If you cannot afford all of the food you consume to be the organic variety, just do the best you can. Take the time to learn which foods retain the most pesticides when grown through conventional methods. In this case, you really are what you eat.

I know you are anxious for me to mention my trusty digestive supplements. I am not here to disappoint, so here goes. Let me start by saying I am not a supplement salesman. I do not take time out of my busy mom life to blog about the lifestyle changes I made in order to take money out of your pocket with some junk supplements that you will take for a while, only to be wearing a size larger than when you first started taking interest in your health. I have been there, done that and I would never wish that misery upon anyone who takes the time to read my work.

The reason I talk about these basic digestive supplements is because *they have changed my life*. If you are wasting time on constant fad diets or you are experiencing menacing health problems, I want to share how the basic supplements can change your life too. Not every person reading this blog will need every supplement I mention, and that is why I am more than happy to provide a personal assessment of what will help you reach your health goals.

## When Science and Poop Collide

The basic components of digestion (breaking down your food) include hydrochloric acid and bile flow. When you begin the chewing motion, your body begins to produce hydrochloric acid in order to break down the food you consume into usable nutrients. Your body was not made to recognize a peanut butter sandwich, so the hydrochloric acid has to break that sandwich down into something your body can recognize as fuel. This is the part of digestion that aids your foods, especially meats and proteins, in not rotting and fermenting in your body. If you have weak acid from various lifestyle choices (poor nutrition or certain medications), the supplement recommended to correct this issue is called Beatine HCL (also referred to as HCL).

The next step of digestion is when your body produces bile to help neutralize the acid. This also helps in effectively removing the unusable nutrients from your body. If your bile is too thick or sticky, this can result in a number of health problems like acne, nausea and gas. The supplement used to correct this issue is called Beet Flow. (Please note, it is very important to always take Beet Flow when supplementing with Beatine HCL to make sure the acid is neutralized properly).

If you have too much hydrochloric acid and not enough bile, this can result in diarrhea. If you do not have enough hydrochloric acid, this can result in constipation. If you do not have enough of either aspect of digestion, well, it results in a big mess that shows up in the form of other health woes and a collection of fat rolls.

The basic digestive supplements I talk about are not meant to be taken for the rest of your life. They are only meant to be taken for as long as your body needs help in restoring proper levels of hydrochloric acid and decent bile flow. How long you need to take them to fix your health problems really depends on how screwed up your current health is.

When I started this program you can see I was pretty screwed up. I *thought* I was healthy because of all of the health shows I watched and weight loss books I devoured. It took me about a year of working really hard on my health before I could finally say my health was improved.

## *My Happily Ever After*

When I first read about the supplements in the <u>*Kick Your Fat in the Nuts*</u> book, I was skeptical to say the least. Thankfully it came at a point in my life where I was desperate enough to try anything to fit into clothing that was not purchased in the maternity section. I could not fathom the thought of becoming the mom who put everyone else's health before herself, resorting to a life of baggy mom jeans and oversized sweaters.

My desperation for real answers turned into a life of optimal health for my entire family. It also made me into a better mom, but not because I can now wear the same size clothes I wore in high school. I no longer need to jump from diet to diet in search of something that can help me lose a few pounds. I no longer have to spend days in bed with my head pounding so hard that I am sometimes unsure if I am having an aneurysm. I now know which foods will help my family flourish and how to prepare those foods instead of giving in blindly to most food companies marketing ploys. Did the supplements do all of this for me? In many ways, yes.

Before I took the steps to improve my <u>digestion</u>, I made valid attempts to eat all of the foods I knew were good for me. I tried really hard. Sometimes it worked, but it was never too long before my old cravings came back and I was hitting the sugar hard.

Despite all of my efforts and the mainstream knowledge I retained over the years, I could not permanently eat the foods I knew were good for my health because of physiological reasons I was unaware of. I truly believe if I did not find these supplements to help improve my digestion, I would still be reading every health book I could while struggling with yo-yoing weight. I believe I would be resorting to the same kinds of medications so many people resort to everyday just to make it through the day. Instead my health is excellent and have more energy than I ever could have imagined.

Does that mean I always pass on my old favorites? Of course not, I am a real human. Since I improved the way my body digests food and have eliminated years of stored toxins, my body is better equipped to handle the occasional splurge. The good news is that occasional splurge does not result in an unstoppable binge or instant weight gain. It is unbelievably freeing. Also, improving my digestion with the natural supplements I mentioned means I do not crave the junk foods any longer. Many times when I do try a food I could previously not live without, it now tastes like cardboard. My body finally recognizes what it needs to thrive and it does not want the food that does nothing for my health.

Digestion is truly the place we all need to start to lose weight and regain our health. While pooping properly may not sound like the key to it all, it is way more important than you would ever imagine. I was on this path of improving my health for at least six months before I truly realized the effect I was having on my body and future health. At first the weight was coming off, and that was all I cared about. Once I realized all of the health improvements I was experiencing as well, it was only then that I finally grasped the pot of gold I stumbled across. Now I want to take what I have learned and pass on that knowledge so my friends and family no longer have to struggle to find real answers.

If you would like to find out more information about how the basic digestive supplements can help you optimize your health, help you lose weight or fix health problems you are dealing with, please do not hesitate to contact me. If you decide to order the supplements from Natural Reference, please use my practitioner code at checkout: nissahelpsme and email me for the instructions on how to properly use them.

# Why So Serious?

Hopefully my quirky sense of humor is coming through in these blogs. I know poop can be a very serious subject, especially if you are unable to poop, but I like funny. Let's all have our good health and enjoy life too!

The next blog *Dear Friend, It's Not Your Fault* takes on a more serious side of this whole weight loss battle. When setting out on a health journey, most people are given some kind of universal plan and then sent on their merry way. There is no individualization to the plans they receive. Guess what that means - high failure rates.

Even the people who manage to successfully lose weight most likely will not keep it off long term. I was in the yo-yo cycle for more than 20 years. IT SUCKS!

The dieter is blamed for not being able to take the weight off and then sent back to an entirely different program with pretty much the same basis - move more, eat less. The dieter fails again and the process repeats.

It's really not the dieter's fault at all. Blame the poopy person who gave you the poopy advice in the first place. There are a lot of poopy people with a lot of poopy advice to go around. Good thing you found this book that is full of good tips; tips that will also help you poop, ironic enough.

# Dear Friend, It's Not Your Fault

Just received another email. Another upset friend blaming herself because she had a bad day. She cheated. She ate junk carbs. She wanted to confess.

## DEAR FRIEND, IT'S NOT YOUR FAULT.

I've been there, far too many times to count. I've done that. So many wasted years: restricting; over exercising; blaming myself when none of it worked.

I struggled. I sweated. I begged. I thought – what if I could just join *The Biggest Loser* – just long enough to lose 30 or 40 pounds. If I could wake up tomorrow with all of this weight magically gone, I promised I would restrict more. I would workout more. I would do whatever it took just to have the weight off for good. I cried. Too many times to count. I wish someone was there to tell me…

## DEAR FRIEND, IT'S NOT YOUR FAULT.

We live in a society that equates being beautiful with being thin. Doctors tell us we need to lose weight to be healthy. Magazines show us workout routines and diets to get us to society's idea of perfection. They all give the same advice – "Count calories. Exercise daily. Eat balanced meals." If you do not lose weight, or when you regain the weight you lost, you are blamed. Once again you are told to eat less, exercise more. More fruits, more vegetables, more healthy whole grains, but eat less of it all.

Many of us have spent years, if not decades, in this exhausting cycle of less food and more exercise. Then we backslide to junk food, couchsurfing and depression over yet another failed diet. When you seek answers regarding what went wrong, the blame comes back to you. You must have eaten too much. You must have not exercised enough. You resolve to start again.

# *DEAR FRIEND, IT'S NOT YOUR FAULT.*

Some are lucky enough to filter through years of bad advice to find real answers. Some of us are able to find diets better suited for our physiology. Diets that remove processed junk (even the foods many consider "healthy"), and diets that add healthy fats that our bodies use for countless functions to <u>thrive</u>.

A ketogenic diet is one of these diets. While some refer to ketogenic diets as restrictive because carbohydrate consumption is often very low, others know a ketogenic diets true power and never feel deprived. They enjoy delicious fats to satiety, while ridding themselves of years of chronic health issues and excess fat that has been around for far too long.

So what about the people who are lucky enough to find a whole food diet like a ketogenic diet, but still struggle? What about the people who see everyone around them having amazing results, yet they cannot stick with this real food diet. I am talking about the people who load up on healthy fats, but still feel weak, sick and ready to give up again.

Is there something wrong with these people that are now "allowed" to eat double bacon cheeseburgers without the bun without the bun every single day, yet they would kill just to eat a large order of fries? Are they broken? Did too many years of restrictive diets doom them once they may have finally found their truth?

What advice do they follow? Eat more fat, but only enough so your body burns its own fat. Eat more protein. Eat less protein. Exercise daily. Relax more. Count calories. Don't pay attention to calories. Even within this narrowed down lifestyle, there is still so much contradictory advice.

## *DEAR FRIEND, IT'S NOT YOUR FAULT.*

If you are following any diet that others claim to be magical, yet you are not getting results, it is time to dig deeper. If you are eating the same foods others see spectacular results with, but you just keep craving the foods you know are not optimal for better health, it is time to end that pattern once and for all. It is time to quit following everyone else's plan that is right for them and find a plan that works for your *bio-individuality*. It is time to make improvements to your body's chemistry so that magical diet becomes magical for you.

Been there. Done that. This time I only have to count to one.

After years of following low fat, then high fat, then no fat, restricted calories, restricted carbs with low fat, Weight Watcher's, Jenny Craig, Slimfast, Atkins...need I go on? After years of trying every diet out there with results that never lasted, is there any wonder our bodies become confused and no longer easily let go of weight? There is a better way to end this lifetime diet mentality and finally take your life back for good.

As humans we are meant to eat whole, real foods and we were never meant to restrict these foods based a fitness app on our phone. Yet that is the plan so many follow. Even with a healthy plan like a ketogenic diet, I still see so many people restricting calories and fat because their phone told them to, instead of listening to what their bodies need. Many of these people are not seeing results long term and will most likely struggle to keep the weight off for good.

Quit struggling. Quit feeling bad. Take your health into your own hands once and for all. Learn how your body works and what foods are optimal for YOU to thrive. Once you invest time into learning this information, life becomes easy.

I searched for more than twenty years for solutions to finally help me with a slew of chronic health conditions. I finally ended more than twenty years of yo-yo diets and chronic poor health. Below are the tips of how you can accomplish the same:

## ALLOW YOUR BODY TIME TO HEAL:

Most likely your body has been abused from years of yo-yo diets, processed foods and over the counter medications to cover up symptoms caused by modern living. **Weight gain is not about eating too many calories and too little exercise.** Weight gain is a symptom of something bigger that is wrong with your body. It could be a chemistry imbalance, a less than stellar digestive system or lifestyle factors like too much stress or too little sleep. Now that you have found a lifestyle full of healing foods, don't expect the weight to fall off overnight. Focus on your health first. Give your body time to heal and then the weight loss will follow.

## FIND YOUR HEALING FOODS:

For some people a keto diet consists of foods high in fat and low in carbs; no other considerations required. Just because someone refers to something as keto does not make it a good choice for you. Test foods with your body. Write down how they make you feel. Monitor your results. Start with a few basic "keto" guidelines and then take the time to figure out *your* perfect keto diet. A diet that makes you feel good and gives you the health results you desire is going to look different for everyone. We are all individuals and have different requirements to help us thrive.

## QUIT EXERCISING TO LOSE WEIGHT:

I didn't say to quit exercising. Exercise is great for mental health and to stay strong well into our senior years. Exercise is *not* great for weight loss. In fact, if you are over exercising, like I did for the majority of my life, this can cause more inflammation and cause your weight to stall. Over exercise just promotes the message of calories in versus calories out. We are eating a keto diet for our hormones, not for caloric restriction. If you keep using exercise as a crutch to eat more of the foods that are not right for you, you will be getting about as far as that treadmill takes you.

Instead of spending many wasted hours sweating on a gym machine, go for a walk a few days per week and find some time to fit in resistance training. This will help you stay healthy and strong. Eating the right foods for your body will help you lose weight.

## FOCUS ON LIFESTYLE:

If you are not sleeping enough to feel well rested or if you are constantly stressed, your body is going to have a difficult time letting go of weight. Everyone has stress – it is a part of life. Sometimes we can't find enough time in the day to sleep. Life gets hard.

How you deal with that stress is key to making a difference in your health and weight loss routine. Quit making excuses about why you cannot get more sleep or reduce your stress. Start implementing small strategies like yoga or meditation to help you destress.

So many people get the wrong message when trying to lose weight. The population as a whole believes the only things we need to do are eat less and move more. Then there is that "smarter", more researched group of people who believe the general population has it all wrong – all you need to do is cut carbs below 20 and the weight will fall off. This is the magic formula to put you into ketosis and now you will live happily ever after. I came here to say *they all have it wrong*.

## LEARN HOW YOUR BODY REALLY WORKS:

This is the one thing the multi-billion dollar health industry does not want you to learn. Once you learn this information, you can take your health into your own hands and you will no longer be a recurring client. Many times when you have trouble sticking to a diet, it is not because you are weak. It is because it is not the right diet for *your* physiology.

Take the time now to learn about how your body digests food and which foods are appropriate for you. Did you know if you commonly have low blood pressure, fasting is not an ideal strategy for you? Did you know if your body is stuck in an anabolic imbalance, eating too much butter and cream can exacerbate this and make weight loss difficult?

So many people in the health industry, even the professionals I trust, give sweeping claims that are meant as advice for everyone. The problem with this is *bio-individuality*. We all thrive with different food sources and different supplements. Quit listening to general claims and trying to make this advice work for you. Invest your resources to figure this out for YOU once and for all.

I obsessed over health and nutrition for over twenty years. I knew nothing until I took the time to learn about my own bio-individuality. Once I learned about myself and followed the advice meant for my specific body chemistry, this all became easy. For the first time in my life, losing weight was not a struggle and I easily maintain it without a second thought.

To finally figure out the correct foods and supplements for you, sign up for this course. Change your life forever.

**DEAR FRIEND,**

I am here to tell you there is *WAY* more to losing weight and regaining optimal health than most professionals will ever tell you. If everyone led you down the right path the first time, the multi-billion dollar health industry would cease to exist.

This path can take time to figure out, but I promise you it is worth it for a life free of caloric restriction and over exercise with little results. If you decide not to take the time to actually learn about yourself and how your body works; if you do not allow your body time to heal before jumping to the next new diet; if you decide to just look for the next quick fix or fast, cheap and general advice meant for everyone, then

# *DEAR FRIEND, IT IS YOUR FAULT.*

# Diet Freedom At Last!

With these next few blogs we are ready to break through conventional diet wisdom to help break you free from diet mentality once and for all. Everything you have been told about diet and exercise up until this book has been lies! LIES! (well, mostly)

Conventional diet programs keep you chained to their purse strings by throwing out tracking and measuring methods that don't even work in the real world. Perhaps some of them might work on a temporary basis...but if they really worked for the long term, why are you here reading yet another diet book?

I mean, I get that I can be funny and perhaps even a little entertaining, but I am guessing you are here for the health and diet jewels of wisdom presented in this book. This means the health and diet jewels of wisdom you received in the past didn't work for you. Why are you still using them?

The next two blogs *Die Scale, Die!* and *Calories, I Wish I Knew How to Quit You* are going to put your diet game down, flip it and reverse it! You are allowed to read the blogs with a bit of skepticism, just as you are allowed to sing that last line in the voice of Missy Elliott.

While we are quoting pop culture, let me say with these next few blogs - don't hate the player, hate the game. You can scream and yell and curse me out all you want. I discovered these truths after more than 20 years of believing the lies myself. Truths they are and nothing you can scream at me will change that.

Now relax a little. Yelling at me raises your cortisol. Raising your cortisol puts you in fat storing mode. I mean, are you even paying attention to these articles?

If you still believe the myths presented over the next few chapters, stop reading for a moment to enroll in my _Coach Me Course_ right now. It will change your life in ways you didn't even know were possible. Plus I use even more bits of pop culture to demonstrate the methods I used to lose weight and keep it off. What other course out there is doing that? Exactly.

# Die Scale, Die!

Who among us doesn't have a case of the Mondays pretty much every single Monday? Being a stay at home mom, pretty much every day is Monday for me, but lately actual Mondays have become so much more Monday-ier.

I am working hard to help people overcome their health issues, while watching their weight fall into place. The problem I continually run into is it seems Monday is torture yourself by stepping on the bathroom scale day. New week, new you! Is that the theory we are all following?

In my yo-yo dieting past, I found the best day to weigh-in was Saturday. Surely I was an angel dieter the entire week, so my efforts were bound to show up on Saturday. This strategy also left me free to indulge on weekend treats. What is up with all of the Monday weigh-ins? Don't you people like to enjoy your weekend properly?

These days I am anti-scale. We had a serious talk, followed by a very dramatic break up. It was pretty much the scene out of *Office Space*, Geto Boys *Die \*MF\* Die* blasting in the background, while I throttled that viscous scale with my toddler's Paw Patrol bat. Man that scale squealed as this suburban mom took out all of her pent up rage during baby nap time.

OK, I just made that up…but it isn't a bad idea. Who doesn't want to smash something so evil with hardcore rap blasting in the background? I just put it away instead. You know, because I am a suburban mom with a napping baby. Crushing that soulless beast who has crushed my spirit so many times before is so not worth waking a sleeping baby.

There is far too much emotion involved with the scale. If you lost weight – wahoo! Time to celebrate. If you gained weight – death, doom and destruction befalls you because the scale went up half a pound. That scale will throw off your entire day. Some people might even go so far as to rethink their entire program just as progress is right around the corner.

If you do see a loss on the scale, there isn't really a reason to celebrate. Sometimes, especially at the beginning of your diet, those pounds you lose could be water weight. Eat half of a sweet potato and boom! Those pounds are coming right back and they will bring a friend or two to the party.

If you gain weight the next week, that could be your blood pressure going up because blood is heavy. This might be a wonderful gain if low blood pressure has become your new BFF. Far too many chronic dieters have low blood pressure and they need extra resources to feel like an actual human.

A scale surplus could be muscle gain accompanying fat loss from the awesome workouts you had this week. Maybe you just need to poop. Are you going to be sad and punish yourself because you have to poop? Embrace your poop. Celebrate your poop. Some people are so constipated, they would commit to watching *Sunny Bunnies* on a never-ending loop just to poop.

You could actually weigh yourself three times in a row and get a different number each and every time. Let's equate the scale to Lindsay Lohan. She is pretty. Everyone wants to believe her when she says she is sober, especially now that she has a British accent. They love her when she flashes that sweet smile, but when she shows up already wasted at the club, look out! Drinks are getting thrown and hair is getting pulled, followed by her new movie getting pulled.

The scale is an undependable liar is the point I am trying to make here. Your scale might even have a British accent to fool you. (If you talk to your scale, I do not have a natural remedy for that.)

## *What That Meanie Scale Really Means*

I could give you the same advice I have been given in the past: when you weigh-in, have no emotion toward the scale. Use it as data. Write it on your spreadsheet and move on with your day.

Right. That will work exactly never. As much as you tell yourself you can weigh-in with no emotion, there is far too much pressure to connect our self worth with the scale in our society.

The problem is the scale is not telling you if you lost or gained fat. The scale is telling you that you lost or gained weight. If you want to lose weight right now, come on over so I can hack off your arm. The rest of your day will probably suck, but hey, the scale said you lost weight. Victory is yours! Now wave your hacked off arm in the air like you just don't care to celebrate your big scale victory!

What if we just ditch the scale all together? What if we go back to connecting with our bodies in the ways of our ancestors? What if we find other ways to pat ourselves on the back other than with our hacked off arm because we were so desperate to see the scale drop that we cut off our arm just to see a loss? I am convinced the scale is really only a lying piece of electronics that is meant to keep us stuck in this awful diet mentality forever.

If you are wondering how the heck you are supposed to measure your results without depending on that lying liar pants on fire scale, check out this excerpt from Day 30 of my _Coach Me Course:_

## *The Scale Still Lies*

*We talked all the way back in week 1 that the scale is a liar. To quote one of my favorite podcastors, "The scale is a lying liar that lies!" If you are still using the scale as your main method to track your progress, just know you are in an abusive relationship with an electronic device that is only telling you one side of the story. It isn't even close to the whole story. It lies. If you like to believe lying liars, keep on keepin on.*

## *Tracking Your Truth*

*If you want to know the truth about how you are progressing with your health journey, this is the way to get to the truth:*

1. *Check in with how you feel. How you feel day to day is the greatest predictor of how healthy you are.*
2. *How do your clothes feel? Are they getting looser? Are they getting tighter? Be honest with yourself.*
3. *Did you measure around your waist this month? How does that compare to your first measurement. If it is down 1/2 - 1 inch, those are wonderful results. What may sound like slow progress is actually wonderful progress!*
4. *Did you take photos of yourself wearing the same outfit you wore last month? Can you see any differences?*

*These are going to be the best ways to track your progress….*

You can take the advice I give to my *Coach Me Course* students on Day 30, apply these tracking methods to your health plan and live happily ever after; or I can lend you my toddler's Paw Patrol bat so you can continually bash yourself in the head with it week after week. Bashing yourself in the head will give you about as much progress as relying on the scale does.

By using these methods to measure progress, your weight and health will advance much further than stepping on the scale. Try it for a month or two, then come back to let me know how much healthier you have become. Or at least come back to read my newest blog.

Now ditch the scale. You will feel so much freedom. Suddenly you will become this diet rebel who doesn't find her worth in a worthless number on the scale. Damn it feels good to be a gangster. Scream it loud and proud – but only if it isn't baby nap time.

If you are still reluctant to let go of the precious scale, check out these side-by-side photos on the next page. Over the holidays I added around ten pounds of happy weight back to my body. After my family vacation in February, I set out on a mission to get back to goal...except the scale didn't move much. When the scale finally did budge, it seemed to go in the wrong direction despite my hard work.

Thankfully I was using other methods to track my progress, such as these photos. My jeans dropped from a size 10, complete with muffin top bulge, to a more relaxed size 6 that glide on. Yet another excellent way to monitor progress.

The scale. It lies. What more proof do you need?

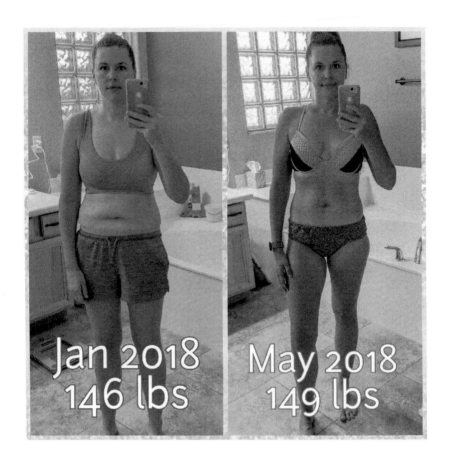

# Calories – I Wish I Knew How To Quit You

Calories in versus calories out. That is the traditional wisdom we all need to get to the bottom of our weight loss woes, correct? If you can workout *really* hard and restrict your calories to what your smartphone app tells you, then you will lose weight. Easy peasy, mystery solved. Let's all pack up and go home – we have calories to count and muffin tops to melt.

Wait a minute. Is this the same weight you have been desperately trying to lose for many years by some method of counting calories? Be it Weight Watchers, Jenny Craig, Nutrisystem, LA Weight Loss, SlimFast, MyFitnessPal or other phone apps – all of these programs work by restricting your calories. So if all of these programs work, why are these companies still in business and why are you still struggling to lose and keep weight off? By George, I think she's onto something!

Let's enter a fairytale world for a second where calories do not matter. This is a world where people eat freely, their bodies function well and they feel great! In this fairytale land, no one has a smartphone telling them how many calories to consume to drop pounds. No one struggles with overexerting themselves on the treadmill. These people are happy and free and have boundless energy. But if the energy runs out, they eat more because they are not counting calories. Doesn't this fairytale sound like an absolute dream world? I like to call this fairytale world *REAL LIFE*.

Can we cut to the chase? Calories in versus calories out only works if you have a calorimeter installed into your body, since that is where this method was derived. A calorimeter is an apparatus for measuring the amount of heat involved in a chemical reaction or other process. Basically it is a flame. Have you had a flame installed into your body? Because if you did I would really like to know about it. My husband is super into technology and this would give us something to talk about other than the color of my youngest son's poop.

I am going to state my very unpopular opinion loud and proud right here. I am going to be hated all around the internet for this opinion. Calorie cultists will shout from the rooftops, "Fat has 9 calories per gram!" They will scream at me that our world would cease to exist if everyone stopped counting calories. I mean, just look at the health of our calorie counting obsessed nation! A nation of true health, that United States of America with all of their fancy calorie counting apps. That is what we all just thought, right?

If this is you, dear calorie cultist, please stop reading. You will not like the things I am about to say. If you want to tell me I am wrong, please be respectable and talk about me behind my back on a Weight Watcher's forum. I work really hard on my articles in order to help people in areas I struggled with for many years. I want you to know stay-at-home moms who write for free for the benefit of others have feelings too. Does anyone know the name of a good support group for abused stay-at-home mom bloggers and the random Internet trolls who shame them?

Alright, here goes! Unpopular opinion alert:

***The amount of calories you eat is not causing you to gain or lose weight.***

Putting that statement in bold and italics means I really mean it.

Calories in versus calories out is just a theory and it is a debunked theory at that. If you are still following the advice of someone telling you to monitor your calories in versus calories out, I have some nifty leg warmers and leotards for you because you are all stuck in the early 80's with your health wisdom. Don't feel bad, so is most of the nation. American Apparel's stock is totally about to go up after everyone reads this blog!

It makes me insane when some poor lost soul is in search of how to lose weight and some former Weight Watchers turned keto diet know-it-all starts spouting out the calories in certain macros and how to manipulate your body into requiring less calories to live a very happy and free life. This happy and free life consists of constantly adding up every last calorie you consume for the rest of your life, along with consistently lowering that amount as time goes on because that is the sustainability of the calories in versus calories out theory. Going lower will never be low enough for very long. When you quit dropping your calories lower, you gain the weight back plus some because you have trained your body to survive on less.

There are approximately 80 calories in a jar of Gerber. I am letting you know this because if you keep following this insane wisdom, that is what you will be eating by the time you are a Golden Girl. If you keep lowering your calories year after year to maintain your weakening metabolism, what's left? That's right, Gerber. Your body will not be able to break anything else down because your metabolism will become so broken and fragile from all of the vitalizing nutrients you have been withholding in the name of calories in versus calories out.

As if hearing someone mention this awful, horrible, outdated calorie advice from random Joe Schmo of the Weight Watcher's world isn't enough, now people in the keto world are trying to make keto and Weight Watcher's collide. They are recommending caloric restriction on a diet based on healing your hormones. They are recommending restricting fat on a high fat diet. Does anyone else not see the problem with any of this? Man I type fast when I'm angry!

## *More Nutrients Help You Heal:*

Eating a ketogenic diet is about healing your hormones. Eating a ketogenic diet is about eating fat. Eating a ketogenic diet is about eating a lot of fat in order to heal your hormones. One of the reasons your hormones are broken is from the constant caloric restriction. What in the Susan Powter is wrong with everybody and their caloric obsession on a diet based on healing hormones by providing your body with nutrients it desperately needs? Did you read that? **Your body needs nutrients to heal, not more restriction of nutrients.**

Now did I just tell you to pound a stick of butter with every meal? No, I did not just tell you to pound a stick of butter with every meal. Please do not accuse me of stuffing our keto friends full of fat like poor foie gras ducks. It is simple – eat fat until you feel good. Satiated is a word I use way too much, but that is what you want. No part of that says to eat everything in your sight because it is fat. No part of that says to stop eating when you are weak, shaky and miserable because your smartphone app told you that you are done with calories today. Just making sure everyone is on the same page here.

If you are restricting your calories, what exactly are you using to heal? Because the few calories you have coming in are going toward breathing. Breathing is important if you want to stay alive. Next, your body might put some of those caloric resources toward growing hair and nails, because people look pretty with hair and nails. If your body is busy using up every last resource you have coming in on basic functions like breathing and growing hair and nails, what is left to heal? Nothing, because you listened to Joe Schmo who graduated from Nutrisystem in 1985. He is now in the process of taking off the same 30 pounds he has been taking off and adding back since 1985. If that's your thing, Joe Schmo it up! If you want to heal and live free of a life of food restriction, put down your dumb smartphone app and listen to me.

## *Been There, Done That:*

If you are still reading, I am going to guess you too counted calories at some point in your life. I am going to guess you too lost weight from counting calories. Hey, so did I! I had success counting calories pretty much every year from 1992 – 2012. Wah-hoo! That's twenty years of calorie counting success!

But that does not mention the failure of always adding back the weight year after year for twenty years – because that happened too. In 2012 I added back the weight plus another 65 pounds on top of that. 65 pounds above my highest weight ever…that is where counting calories got me. Oh, and a fast track to diabetes. Forgot that part as well.

Right. That's the part Jenny Craig fails to mention when Kirstie Alley flaunts her swimsuit figure on Oprah. When Kirstie gained the weight back, it was Valerie Bertinelli's turn. But then Jenny Craig had to ditch both of them because the weight came back. And then Kirstie lost the weight again, which was great for Jenny Craig because no one seemed to care that she is a lifelong yo-yo dieter from caloric restriction – they just see a skinny Kirstie Alley on their television. Well, until Jenny Craig hides her again because the weight comes back.

People like to ooh and aah at the magic caloric restriction brings, but what about the struggle to maintain that loss? Suddenly those turn into "Woah, what happened?" kinds of ooh's and aah's. Much different ooh's and aah's.

So if caloric restriction doesn't work for Jenny Craig, if it doesn't work for Weight Watchers and if it didn't work for me after twenty years of type-A personality attempts, why is everyone trying so hard to make it work with keto?

## *But My Friend Lost Weight Counting Calories:*

Surely someone is having success with counting calories since it is all the rage.

There *are* reasons restricting your calories might work; however, this will only work for a little while until you have to restrict even further. When most people start counting calories, they take the time to pay attention and write down what they eat. This means most likely they will skip Dunkin Donuts in the morning and opt for something not so high in calories, like bacon and eggs. What is the difference there? Bacon and eggs are both real foods. They are made up of components your body can recognize and use as fuel instead of junky, processed carbohydrates that your body has no idea what to do with. These junky carbs will be stored as toxic fat. The bacon and eggs will break down more appropriately to give you energy.

More real food and less processed junk leads to health improvements and weight loss. The bacon and eggs person's insulin will not spike as high because of the foods chosen. This gives the body the opportunity to burn fat once the insulin levels out. This is hormonal and not caloric.

If you take two people who eat 500 calories every day for breakfast, but one eats donuts and the other eats bacon and eggs, which one is going to have an easier time losing weight? Right, the bacon and eggs person because bacon and eggs do not spike insulin as high as donuts. Same calories, but one person was smart and ate a breakfast to heal her hormones and satiate her longer. Let's call that smart girl Nissa. (You can rename the smart girl when you write your article).

Now if our smart girl Nissa keeps her insulin low all day by eating appropriate food for her hormones that do not cause large insulin spikes, smart Nissa can eat as much food as she needs to feel satiated with nary a calorie counted. She keeps her insulin low, she feels good, she does not feel like a mad scientist adding up calories and macros all day, and she loses weight with ease. This also takes into account that smart Nissa chooses appropriate foods her body can digest, that also keep her insulin spikes low and infrequent. This will be different for everyone, but smart Nissa has taken the time to learn what her body can and cannot <u>digest</u> through trial and error.

Now let's say smart Nissa steps onto the scale on Monday morning. Smart Nissa sees the weight on the scale went up by one pound. Smart Nissa's mind is thrown into a tizzy and she panics! She determines the diet that has been making her feel great and helping her lose clothing sizes is no longer working because an electronic device with absolutely no connection to how she feels told her she gained one pound. Smart Nissa decides to take advice from Joe Schmo and starts restricting her calories on a diet based on hormones.

Smart Nissa is no longer smart because before she restricted her calories, her body was getting the resources it needed to heal and balance out her hormones. Now that she is restricting her calories based on her smartphone app's recommendations, previously smart Nissa's body starts to go into famine mode because barely enough nutrients are coming in for even the most basic of functions. Previously smart Nissa's body is going to hold onto every ounce of stored fat because her body will need that as more and more nutrients are restricted. Smart Nissa's body will start breaking down her lean muscle mass to make up for the lack of nutrients coming in. Her formerly well functioning metabolism is being lowered. Now smart Nissa will have to eat even less to lose weight or simply maintain the loss.

## *The Reality of Calorie Restriction:*

My favorite podcaster TC Hale says it best – you cannot pay 1800 dollars worth of bills with only 900 dollars of income. You may get by for a month or two with this tight budget, but eventually Froylan from *Operation Repo* will come calling. I mean, everyone wants to be on TV, but those people are scary! Maybe just pay your car note and try out for *America's Got Talent* instead. You don't even need real talent to have Simon call you names!

In our case, you cannot use 1800 calories of nutrients required just to function with only taking in 900 calories. Something somewhere will need to be cut. Is it lean muscle mass you need for a stronger metabolism? Will hair begin falling out of your head at an alarming rate because you do not have the proper resources to keep it attached? Will you go through depression, anxiety and hormonal imbalance fits of rage lashing out at your family because you are so starved of nutrients? Yes. Yes. Yes.

Your body needs to conserve that energy somewhere and it will never be the functions you require to live. Your body will steal the resources it no longer has coming in from other areas of your body, like muscle mass or healthy hair growth. Then your metabolism slows down even more. This means you will have to keep lowering the amount of nutrition you are taking in just to maintain the weight loss.

At some point this becomes completely unsustainable if you want to stay alive.  Add obsessive exercise to the mix and holy body freak out. Your body panics and goes directly into famine mode. When you are in famine mode for many years, like many people are, your body just starts ceasing functions that previously were fine tuned. I cannot say that caloric restriction is the reason for all of our health problems, but it is definitely a contender.

Some of the healthiest people on Earth do not understand how calories work. They eat real, whole foods when they are hungry and they stop when they are full. They listen to their bodies and easily maintain their weight and health. It is when our crazy westernized methods of controlling every little aspect of life with our smart apps infiltrates them, or when they start eating our one hundred calorie snack packs instead of an apple – that is when the problem starts.

Even after all of this, people are still going to throw tomatoes at me and tell me I am leading people astray. There is just no possible way you can lose weight going through life based on how your body feels rather than tracking your calories with an app. You *need* technology to tell you what to do! That's just the way our society works. No one in the history of our human race has ever successfully lost weight while not tracking their calories.

## *My Big Fat Calorie Life Story:*

My entire life I tracked calories because that is what I was told to do. Like a good girl, I limited my calories to somewhere around 1200 per day. I exercised 1-2 hours per day, at least five days per week. This is what all of the websites and diet companies said someone of my height and weight required to lose weight. This is what I looked like most of that time:

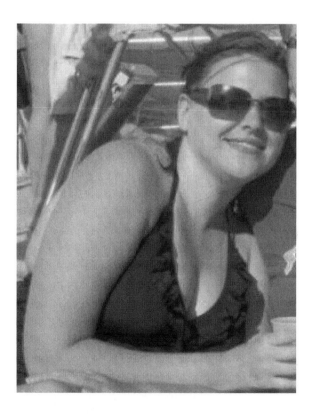

In 2013 I finally came to my senses and stopped tracking calories. I finally did the work to tune in with my body and ate based on how I feel. I stopped looking to technology to tell me how my body feels, and started looking to my body to tell me how my body feels. Now I live a life free of caloric restriction and mad scientist tracking methods. If I am hungry, I eat. If I am full, I stop. Now it really is easy peasy, mystery solved.

Please tell me this. If counting calories on a diet based on hormones is still the only way to lose weight, how have I lost a total of 145 pounds and kept it off with minimal effort without counting one calorie? And when I do take the time to add up a day's worth of food for sake of demonstration, how is it that I now eat 2200-2400 calories daily when every calorie tracker on Earth tells me I need to limit my caloric intake to only 1200-1300 with an hour plus of cardio to maintain my weight? How is this all possible if I am wrong? Am I some strange alien being whose previous life of restriction no longer applies because I am suddenly magic?

This works for my husband too. He doesn't count calories or limit his fat. He is down 80 pounds this year. Oh, and there are my clients who I tell to eat more since most of them eat meals fit for birds. They add more food and once their hormones begin to heal, they lose weight too. Are we all just witch doctors? Or did we just stop listening to all of the experts and media who want to take our money by keeping us on this constant diet hamster wheel?

## *The Calories In vs. Calories Out Winners:*

Who else does calories in versus calories out benefit more than the health or food and beverage industries? If health companies can convince you to eat their junk processed meal bars to lose weight because they fit into your calorie budget; if trainers can convince you that working out with them just a little bit more can help you reach your health goals; if soda companies can convince you that you need to move a little bit more to burn that Coke you just drank, or better yet, that the Diet Coke has zero calories, therefore zero impact on your waistline; if they can keep you convinced, they can keep you on the hamster wheel and keep the money coming to them. I chose to stop giving them my money a few years ago and it has never been easier to maintain a healthy lifestyle at my ideal weight.

If you insist that counting calories is the only way, I have absolutely no problem with this. In the famous words of Nene Leakes – you do you boo. When you gain the weight back next year, this blog will still be here. Come back if you are ready; or try counting calories *again*.

If you do not want to believe me because you think I am just some Joe Schmo on the Internet, some of the smartest people in the industry are spreading the same message – TC Hale, Leanne Vogel, Shawn Mynar, Jimmy Moore, Doc Nally. They all teach to eat for your hormones. Are they all witch doctors too?

# Advanced Methods

Now that your head is spinning, we are really going to get into the good stuff! I understand that it might take some time to come to grips with these previous dieting jewels all being big fat liar, liar pants on fires, so take your time with that. Go back and read the blogs again for clarification. Let the truth sink in.

With these next two articles *You Don't Got Ketones, Brah!* and my new *Filthy Fast Plan* we are going to get into more advanced topics of ketosis and some advanced techniques of intermittent fasting. If you aren't quite ready for the advanced topics yet, no fear. Read for the funny and proceed only when you are up for the challenge.

Also, be excited! The *Filthy Fast Plan* is new and only available to readers of this book and students of my *Coach Me Course: Escape Diet Mentality and End Yo-Yo Diets Forever.* This is the course where I spend six weeks really getting into the nitty gritty of the daily tricks I used to shed the fat and easily maintain that loss for the first time in my life! It is also another way to help you get ready for these more advanced techniques since I take the time to walk you through how I prepared myself. Believe it or not, I was once a beginner too!

If you are enjoying this book, you would definitely enjoy the course - it is a full six weeks of my humorous, yet educational, health musings combined with six weeks of motivational videos and ten full guides to get you started on the right track with your low-carb, high-fat lifestyle. (Many of those also entertain combined with maximum health education).

On a separate note, the *Filthy Fast Plan* came about this past spring when I desperately needed to look good in a bikini since I was about to be photographed in my first bikini ever for more than

3 million readers in *People Magazine!* That's right...my first public bikini display in my life was in a national magazine. Yes, that is as scary as it sounds. My plan to get into tip top bikini shape had to be good and now it is all written out for you to give it a try!

PS...if you haven't had a chance to read my feature article in *People Magazine,* check it out here.

# *You Don't Got Ketones, Brah!*

Recently I am on the receiving end of several distraught messages from various women stating they are doing everything right with their ketogenic diet, but their weight loss has either stalled or reversed directions. They send me their food logs…their measly, scrappy food logs filled with dry chicken breasts and iceberg salad combos with barely a lick of salad dressing. When I ask them where's the fat, they insist someone on the keto boards told them to not eat fat so they can burn their own body fat.

Seriously, I want to shake them. I want to shake them and their misinformed message board counterparts and scream. My inner Mike 'The Situation' Sorrentino comes out as I emotionally pump my fist and yell, "You don't got ketones, brah!" Good thing all of these exchanges are via email so no one actually witnesses my fist pumping rage.

I typically reply more politely by letting them know if they are eating like a sorority girl trying to fit into a formal dress, they do not have ketones and typically a ketogenic diet is not effective without ketones.

Ninety-nine percent... Wait, scratch that. One hundred percent of the time I receive a follow up email insisting they are in ketosis because their pee sticks turned purple. For the love of all things gym-tan-laundry can we please dump those urine strips wherever Pauly D stores his hair gel? Because his hairstyle doesn't even make sense and neither do your precious pee sticks.

<u>Testing for blood ketones</u> is expensive, I get it. Why pay the big bucks for the only reliable way to test for ketones when you can get urine on your hands and have a pretty purple pee stick picture to flash on the message boards? Well, I think I just answered that. Testing for ketones with a blood ketone monitor is the only reliable way to know if you are in ketosis.

The urine strips you are using are most likely indicating you are dehydrated. They *may* have a touch of validity at the very beginning as your body begins excreting ketones through urine (also called acetones), but if you are in true ketosis those strips do not work very long since your ketones will soon only be detectable via blood (beta-hydroxybutyrate). I was going to make a female time of the month joke here, but that would be gross. So is peeing all over your hands, by the way.

For those people who just want to wing it and hope for the best, there are better ways of guessing if you are in ketosis. I will chit chat with you about them below. If you have never watched *Jersey Shore*, you might hate this blog.

**If when you wake up the first thing you do, after testing your urine ketones, is jolt to the kitchen to scarf down last night's pizza that was left on the counter, YOU DON'T GOT KETONES, BRAH!**

Most people powered by ketones are not typically hungry first thing in the morning, so there is no racing to the kitchen for food. Many don't even require coffee right away because of the energy and mental clarity provided by burning ketones. Many who follow a ketogenic diet also naturally fall into an intermittent fasting routine which helps you stay in ketosis, along with many other health benefits.

I have been in ketosis for quite some time and my typical first meal falls somewhere between 10 am – 12 pm. This is not because I am trying to fast, but because I am busy and that is the first time I even think about food. Your brain becomes more focused on other tasks when it is not constantly searching for glucose to burn. My brain focuses on getting two kids fed and keeping them from killing each other until sweet baby nap time relief. If I was a glucose burner and had to stop to make myself breakfast, surely one kid would have carpet marks permanently wedged onto his face by now from being held down by the other while fighting over a plastic shovel from the dollar store.

*If lunch just ended and all you can do is daydream about the tacos you are not allowing yourself for dinner, YOU DON'T GOT KETONES, BRAH!*

When you are burning fat as fuel, you will naturally crave more fat since your body now realizes fats true value in keeping you satiated. If all you can do is think about the carbs you cannot have, your body hasn't switched over to using fat as fuel. You need to increase the amount of fat you eat at each meal substantially to help your body switch modes.

As mentioned above, fat burners brains are too busy solving the mysteries of quantum mechanics than to sit and daydream about food. (Wow, I sure make us Ketonians sound smart. I really have no idea what that sentence means. It sounded smart).

*If you are shoving protein shakes and protein bars down your throat every two to three hours, YOU DON'T GOT KETONES, BRAH!*

When you are a fat burner, you can literally go days without a meal. Sometimes you will go an entire day and realize you actually forgot to eat. When you are a glucose burner, you have whatever you recently ate to burn before your body requires more energy. When you are a fat burner, you tap into all of that stored energy you have been conserving overtime. If you can't make it from one meal to the next, or even skip a meal every now and then without getting hangry, you, my friend, are not a fat burner.

*If you are walking to the Shore Store and get ravenous at the smell of fried elephant ears, YOU DON'T GOT KETONES, BRAH!*

Most fat burners can take in the smell and keep strutting down the shore. It may even make some fat burners gag a little remembering how that junk made them feel back in their glucose burning days. Tired, lethargic, fat. Who needs it, bro? If you are ravenous or have a strong desire for carbs in between meals, start eating more satiating fats with your meals.

If that doesn't work, check in with your digestion to make sure your body is actually using the foods you are eating. If you are eating a lot of high quality fat but still craving carbs, or worse – gaining weight, you are most likely not digesting those high quality fats correctly.

***If right before the G in GTL you feel the need to have a banana or protein shake like many fitness professionals recommend, YOU DON'T GOT KETONES, BRAH!***

When you are fat fueled, you are literally fueled by fat. The fat on your body is usually enough to push you through most workouts. Fasted weight lifting is more effective because your human growth hormone (HGH) levels are higher when lifting fasted. Higher HGH means much quicker results with less time spent in the gym. If you partake in cardio workouts, these are better fasted too. Instead of burning the glucose you just ate, you will burn stored body fat. I think that's kind of the point.

If you require meals right before or directly after your workouts, you still have work to do before becoming fat adapted. Maybe ditch the gym and get into the kitchen to make some fat bombs first. Food always trumps workouts when it comes to weight loss. Repeat that one hundred times if you still do not believe it. Let it sink in a little.

***If you prefer to watch a Snooki and Jwoww marathon because you are just too exhausted to make it to the Shore Store to pretend to sell t-shirts, YOU DON'T GOT KETONES, BRAH!***

When you are truly in ketosis, it's almost shocking how much energy you have. When I first began a ketogenic diet, I couldn't even sit still to watch an episode on my precious *The Real*

*Housewives*. I had this overwhelming urge to vacuum the floors. And then I had to have clean counters. Wait, there was a spot on the windows; I had to wipe them again. WHO WAS I? I had been a couch potato for most of my life and suddenly I became Molly Maid when my baby was napping. In my only time to relax I had copious amounts of energy to do anything but relax!

When I was a glucose burner, all I dreamed of all day long was throwing my feet up and watching the dvr with a huge bowl of microwave popcorn. And that is pretty much what I did with any ounce of spare time. With ketones, I have a clean house! Ok, that's a lie. I have two kids under 4 years old which means I have pretzel crumbs and legos covering every square inch of my house. But you best believe I am constantly picking those things up instead of sitting on my butt studying how Doc McStuffins saves the day. Instead I walk around the house, hands full of legos while humming about taking ouchies away. So. Much. Better.

***If someone isn't currently explaining to you that they are not eating fat on a ketogenic diet in order to burn their own body fat and you still have the negative attitude of Mike 'The Situation' Sorrentino, YOU DON'T GOT KETONES, BRAH!***

When your brain is busy burning ketones, the world suddenly becomes a very happy place. You start to notice all of the birds singing and the flowers dancing and your husband's chewing may even become cute when it once made you want to rip all of his teeth out one by one.

OK, that one went too far for this girl with a slight case of misophonia. Ketones are wonderful. Ketones are great. Ketones are not miracles. But you get the picture. Ketones make you happy! Ketones turn you into Mary Poppins, but without the spoonful of sugar because, you know – ketones.

If you are burning fat as fuel appropriately, your day should not be filled with mood swings or constant crashes that are often felt by sugar burners. Your brain fog clears and your thoughts become lighter, clearer and more concise. You develop a better, happier attitude in life. There is a pep in your step and gratitude in your heart. Then again, why shouldn't there be? You have created this healthy life for yourself with unlimited amounts of energy and copious food intake. When you are burning ketones, you get to eat lots of delicious food! No more starving yourself. No more killing yourself at the gym. Life becomes easy. How can anyone be mood swingy about that?

I want everyone reading this to have ketones, brah, but in a less muscle meathead kind of way. The best way and only way to know for sure is to test with your blood monitor. The strips are expensive, but even just testing once or twice per week will give you a better indication than guessing with urine strips. Finally figuring out if you are for sure in ketosis will give you a better idea of what you need to do to stay there.

Simply dropping your carbs below 20 and adding a little fat to your diet isn't enough for most people. For some people that may work, but for others there are more steps you can take to get there. But you do not know if you need to take those steps unless you know where your *ketones are registering*.

Also know that switching from a lifelong glucose burner to a fat burner does not happen overnight. Quit expecting to change your lifetime habits for just one day, then waiting for a miracle to happen. It could take a week. It could take multiple weeks. It really could take much longer if you are not testing and have no clue if what you are doing is working.

The point is, you need to give this process time. You need to give your body time to figure out how to switch to this optimal fat burning mode. If you are rushing the process in despair, you will never know just how amazing this life can be.

If you *have* been patient; if you have done everything I talked about and you are still feeling the steroid rage felt by our Jersey

Shore friends, there are things you can do to speed along the fat burning process:

1. **Add more fat to your diet.** Typically when someone comes to me and is not losing weight on a ketogenic diet, the answer is usually add more fat. Eating a low calorie diet full of fat is still a low calorie diet. Low calorie diets can raise your insulin, which is the opposite of a ketogenic diet's purpose. Try adding more fat – see if that helps you. It's kind of like when you ask IT for help. They always ask if you restarted your computer. Let's equate adding more fat to restarting your computer.
2. **Give intermittent fasting a try:** The process of fasting really can kick a body into ketosis faster. Even just an overnight fast of 12-14 hours is helpful for some people. If your body is really stubborn, you may need to work on your fasting muscle and stretch it for longer periods of time.
3. **Digestion, digestion, digestion:** A ketogenic diet can be a miracle for anyone, but should not be attempted immediately by everyone. If your body is not digesting protein or fat well, your body will really hate you when you take away it's precious processed carbohydrates. It will hate you in the form of burning diarrhea. It will hate you in the form of baseball sized constipation. It will hate you in the form of oily zits all over your pretty little face. If you are experiencing poor digestion in any form when switching to a ketogenic diet, it would be wise to take a step back and work on your digestion. If you don't, your body will continue to store your food as toxins. This means you stay fat and miserable. If you are interested in learning more about digestion, start with the almost free digestion course found here.
4. **Work with a coach:** I hate to toot my own horn as much as I hate that phrase, but I have helped many people get on their merry ketone way. If you are really struggling, give coaching a try. There is way more to this health stuff than you may have time to research, so hiring someone who has already done the research can move things along and keep you motivated to continue. When you continue, you reach your goals. People I work with are making new strides

everyday – hitting goal weights they haven't seen in years and improving health markers in ways even working with their doctor did not improve. This stuff works, but only if you do it right and stick with it.

Also, I will say this every time – my information is educational, not medical advice. Listen to your doctor. If your doctor does not stay updated on health topics, find a new doctor. Always continue to educate yourself as well.

I was really struggling with a clever way to end this blog. I looked down and realized the majority of the time I spent writing this blog I have been wearing a white 'wife beater' tank top that says 'Husband Beater.' (Don't report me to PETA or whoever takes up abused spousal cases. It's a joke. My husband is twice my size. I don't beat him). I am not sure if the shirt inspired the blog or the blog inspired the shirt. I do know Mike 'The Situation' Sorrentino just helped me explain ketones to you, and that is something I never thought would happen. Miracles. Miracles everyday, people.

# How I Dropped from Size 10 to Size 6 in Less than Six Weeks!

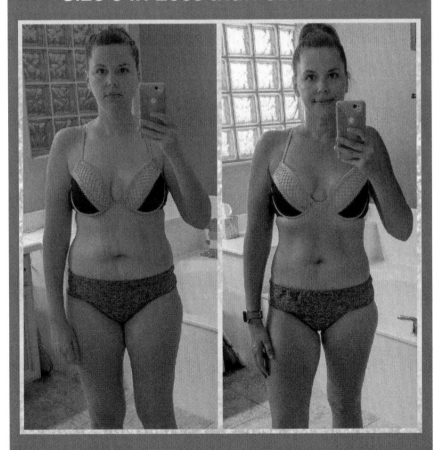

Nissa Graun:
@eatingfatisthenewskinny

# Filthy Fast Plan

## How I Dropped from a size 10 to a size 6 in less than six weeks

Let me start out by stating I am not a fan of crash diets. I watched *Saved By The Bell* religiously as a kid. I still vividly remember the episode where Jessie Spano used caffeine pills to keep up with her academics and the exercise videos she was filming. In the very next scene, she collapsed into Zach Morris' arms crying out, "I'm so excited. I'm so excited. I'm so...scared." The drama those tween shows provide can leave a lasting impact.

That's not to say I never tried to lose weight quickly or even tested out those kinds of pills that are advertised as safe, but in reality do horrible things to your body. I just did those things in secret. I think I kept it all a secret because I didn't want anyone to talk me out of the awful decision I was making out of pure desperation to get thinner.

Everytime I started what some might consider to be a crash diet, thankfully I never lasted long enough for it really to affect my health. I was weak and my junk food addiction was strong. End of story.

When I finally succeeded at taking the weight off for good, I realized all of those quick fix gimmicks are a scam and not meant for lasting weight loss or better health. I improved my digestion and corrected my chemistry, which made it so easy to change my eating habits to the way I plan to eat for life - delicious, fatty, real foods.

This past March when I received a message that *People Magazine* wanted to include me in their feature 100 pounds down article, I was absolutely on cloud nine...until I got the email that it would be a bathing suit edition. My body was still trying to find it's happy weight after losing more than 100 pounds, so I was a little less than swimsuit ready. I will also admit I did slack off a little over the holidays and during our post holiday family vacation to Disneyland. I mean, it's the happiest place on Earth and I never even tried a churro before. Disneyland has churros everywhere. You get where I am going here...

I don't view taking occasional breaks from eating a low-carb, high-fat diet as a failure. This is going to be my lifestyle forever. If I want to make it work, sometimes I need to taste new delicacies, if you consider churros a delicacy. At the same time, I needed to get back into swimsuit shape well before swimsuit season was upon us.

To get swimsuit ready, I started to cut back my carbs from my maintenance level of 50-80 per day to more like 30-50 per day. That is what works for my body and the level where I feel best. I also made sure to only eat in an eight hour window each day, which wasn't too difficult since I already did that most days anyway. Ever since I started daily intermittent fasting, that schedule has become my norm. I knew sticking to that routine would help the weight come off slowly and steadily.

The dilemma I faced is I had a deadline. I was being considered for a swimsuit edition of a national magazine with more than 3 million copies printed each week. Slow and steady wasn't going to cut it for me this time. Luckily I also know myself well and knew any type of crash diet to lose the weight quickly would just make me feel bad and damage my metabolism. I needed to figure out a plan where I could still feel great every day, while also shedding fat at a quicker than normal pace for my body.

## *How the Filthy Fast Plan came to be:*

After gaining a little bit of winter weight over the holidays, I got back to researching the best method to lose the stubborn regained pounds. Basically I was lazy and didn't want to count carbs, so I was looking for an easier way. At this time I was really into researching different fasting methods. I followed some of the methods talked about in my favorite new fasting group with less than impressive results.

Even though I wasted precious time that could have been spent preparing for my bikini shoot, I did take away a valuable lesson from the experience. Just because a lot of people rave about a method working for them, it doesn't mean it will work for you. Everyone is coming from a different place metabolically, so they need different programs. Eating one meal each day, while relaxing my carb count to non-keto levels, is not in my metabolic profile; not to lose weight anyway.

The same thing goes for this program. Is this filthy fasting plan guaranteed to work for you just because I had such awesome results? Nope, absolutely not.

If you test it out, feel good on the program and give your body enough time to adapt, will it most likely work? Probably. It is the fastest and easiest method I have tried and if I was able to get such amazing results with already being so close to my goal, it will most likely work for someone who has a little extra weight to lose and who isn't in such a hurry.

I also want to remind you while you will most likely lose body fat at a quicker pace with this method, those efforts may not show up on the scale. Remember - I lost two entire pants sizes and gained three pounds in this six week period. ***The weight gained was not fat.*** With fasting and a little bit of work in the gym, I gained bone density and muscle while losing fat. All big wins!

When I was searching through my new fasting group, I saw a woman who was having amazing results with alternate day fasting three days per week. What this plan entails is three 36 hour fasts every week, falling on alternate days.

An example of this would be:

- Eat dinner Sunday
- Start fast at 7 pm Sunday night and do not eat anything all day Monday.
- Resume a twelve hour eating window on Tuesday at 7am and eat until Tuesday at 7pm.
- Continue this routine throughout the week until you have 3 full fast days combined with 4 full feasting days.

While I wasn't super excited about not eating for three entire days each week, her results were amazing and I had a tight deadline, so I decided to give it a try. After all, last year I was doing a few 24 hour fasts each week to get to my goal; how much harder could it be to go a little longer... especially if I was sleeping most of that time?

One night. I lasted one night on this plan before I gave it up.

It's not that it is really all that much harder than a 24 hour fast; it's just that it was too much fasting for my situation at the time.

First of all, while my body was trained to fast 16 hours each day, it had been a while since I practiced the longer fasts. When I previously did 1-2 24 hour fasts per week to get to my goal, I worked up to that. With my approaching deadline, I didn't really have the time to work up to it.

Also, my husband travels a lot for work while I take care of two young kids. They are really cute; at least until they argue over toys all day, push each other off the couch and won't eat a single thing I make them for dinner. By 5 pm I am ready to let my husband take over so I can relax by cooking dinner and washing the dishes. (If only my twenty something year old self could hear me now - I said washing dishes is how I relax).

My point here is, while I could probably have completed the three 36 hour fasts that gave this other girl such fabulous results, I was too stressed out to give that plan much effort. As you learned in previous lessons, stress does not help us achieve our goals.

Finally, I like to eat. Plain and simple. Not eating three days each week made me feel a little anorexic. To be frank, a lot of people live this lifestyle and it is not anorexic at all. In fact, many great health benefits can come from a plan like alternate day fasting...it just isn't right for me. It is a little too much restriction to float my fasting boat. I eat a low-carb, high-fat diet with daily fasting because I no longer want to feel restricted. That is the reason I made the choice to find a happy medium and create my own *Filthy Fast Plan* - a plan that could help me speed up progress without feeling restricted.

Here is how the plan I followed works:

# *The Filthy Fast Plan*

- You will eat your normal keto or low-carb, high-fat plan to satiety four days each week. Eat to satiety and do not restrict calories these days.
- You will eat according to the *Filthy Fast Plan* three days per week
- This plan works best if you alternate the days, but do not stress about it too much when you have back to back filthy fast days or back to back feasting days.

So what do I mean by a filthy fast day? If you read the basic fasting guide already (which I hope you have since this is a more advanced plan), you will know I advocate for a clean fast. This means no food, caloric drinks or artificial sweeteners outside of your designated eating window. On a filthy fast day you should still adhere to that rule for as long as you can tolerate. If that means 14 hours for you, great! If that means 18 hours with no food, even better! The longer you can go without feeling unwell or overly hungry, the better.

Your best results will come from this filthy fast plan if you can consume all of your food in one or two meals on a filthy fast day...or even a few snacks, followed by a bigger meal. At the beginning stick to what works for you and add more fasting only as you feel ready.

Once you decide you are ready to eat, you will follow what some call a fat fast for the remainder of the day. Do your best to make 80-90% of the calories you eat on a filthy fast day calories from fat. The next highest macro you consume that day will come from protein. Do your best to consume very low carbs on a filthy fast day. If you consume under 20-30 grams, you should be good.

## So what can you eat on a fat fast?

My favorite thing to eat early in the day is fat bombs. I focus on fat bombs without artificial sweeteners and fat bombs lower in carbs. I also like coconut oil based fat bombs because they really prep your body to burn fat. I will typically eat a handful of fat bombs around noon and then another handful around 3. That keeps me feeling good until dinner.

If fat bombs are not your thing, a bulletproof coffee with no artificial sweetener can work well too.

For dinner I typically eat whatever I feel like that day as far as meats and veggies are concerned. I measure the portions on my food scale so I do not go overboard on the calories taken in on a filthy fast day. More about that below.

There are many other options you can choose on a filthy fast day. Google "fat fast" and you will find plenty of delicious options like bacon and eggs cooked in butter or salads with avocados and creamy dressings. Think of some of your own favorite high-fat foods and mix it up. Or stick to the simple fat bomb plan like me.

To be honest, part of the reason I enjoy the filthy fast days is that I can just grab fat bombs until dinner; no extra meal prep required. This saves a lot of meal prep and clean up time for this busy mom.

## 3 More Filthy Fast Rules

**The second rule** is you should keep the calories you consume lower than your feasting days. Try to eat somewhere between 1,000 - 1200 calories on the filthy fast days. This plan is the only time I will tell you to pay attention to calories. I will explain why in a moment. If you eat a little over or under your allotment, no big deal. Just do your best to keep your calorie intake on the low end on filthy fast days.

**The third rule** for a filthy fast day is to eat in a shorter window than you are accustomed to. So if you typically eat 16:8, where you fast for 16 hours and eat only in an 8 hour window, try to push your fast even longer to complete an **18:6 fast** or a **20:4** fast. Only push yourself over time as you feel ready. Remember, this is for the filthy fast days only for this plan. You should still eat on your normal schedule the other 4 days each week.

The longer you can fast, the longer your body is burning fat, so do your best to keep your fast going on filthy fast days. Since you will be eating mostly fat, your insulin levels will remain low, so eat when you feel you are ready. Figure out the right balance for your situation.

**The fourth rule** for the filthy fast is to **make sure you eat on your feasting days**. While I never want you to force food beyond satiety, part of the reason this plan works so well is it revs your metabolism up by taking in various amounts of calories each day. Basically by keeping your body guessing about what is coming in that day, you are going to stoke your overall metabolic burn. It is important to have higher calorie days mixed with lower calorie days. This is also called cycling your calories.

Without having to go too overboard with counting calories, this is an example of cycling your nutrient intake for a greater metabolic burn rate:

# Filthy Fast Cycling Example:

**Sunday:** normal plan: approximately 2,000 calories consumed over 8-10 hour period

**Monday: FFD:** approximately 1,000 calories consumed after 1 pm, consisting mostly of fat. Stop eating by 6 pm.

**Tuesday:** normal plan: approximately 2,200 calories consumed over 8-10 hour period

**Wednesday: FFD:** approximately 1,200 calories consumed after 1 pm, consisting mostly of fat. Stop eating by 6 pm.

**Thursday:** normal plan: approximately 2,100 calories consumed consumed over 8-10 hour period

**Friday: FFD:** approximately 1,100 calories consumed after 1 pm, consisting mostly of fat. Stop eating by 6 pm.

**Saturday:** normal plan: approximately 2,000 calories consumed consumed over 8-10 hour period

## *My Typical Filthy Fast Day:*

Clean fast until noon. Only water or black coffee.
**12 pm:** 5 minty melts with water
**3 pm:** 3 minty melts and 1 chocolate butter with water
**5 pm:** 4 oz marinated steak, ½ pan Coconut Cauliflower Fried Rice with water
*Drink water and take sea salt under tongue throughout the day to stay hydrated*

Fast until 10 am the next day.

Is that exactly 1,000 - 1200 calories on a filthy fast day? I cannot be exactly sure since I don't always measure ingredients when I cook, but it is close enough for my purpose here. As long as I am mixing it up most days of the week, that is close enough for my body to respond.

I am also feasting to satiety on the other 4 days of the week. I am sure to never restrict calories on those days. I eat according to my normal low-carb, high-fat schedule until I feel good, but not too stuffed.

## *Strategies Utilized in the Filthy Fast Plan:*

- *Fat Fast:* Eating 80-90% of your calories from fat on filthy fast days

- **_Calorie Cycling:_** Having low calorie days mixed with high calorie days
- **_Fasting Mimicking:_** Tricking your body into believing you are fasting with low calorie days that have low insulin spikes due to high fat intake
- **_Fast Cycling:_** Alternating days of longer periods of fasting with days of feasting

This is the plan I developed when I needed to drop fat quickly for my upcoming photoshoot. Please notice how I said fat and not weight. I actually gained three pounds over the six week period, but you can definitely see fat loss in the photos even with a higher number on the scale.

If I thought of this plan sooner, I would have used this plan intermittently while trying to get to my original goal weight. It is a great plan to keep your body guessing and the fat loss coming.

I would advise to take breaks from this plan every six weeks or so just to mix things up and ensure you are not being too restrictive with your fasting. Always remember to listen to your body. This plan is another tool in getting to your weight loss and health goals, however it is not necessary to hit your goals if it does not feel right for you.

# More Healing, Less Work

Woo hoo! Are you ready to get out there and start shedding all that fat? Well, I guess there is really nowhere to go and not much to do unless you plan to grocery shop for some healing foods. Seriously. Your fat shedding is going to come from the food you eat, not so much from the exercise aspect that has been drilled into your head by shows like *The Biggest Loser*. Have you seen most of those contestants lately? Look them up. Many are sadly back to where they started.

If you haven't figured it out by now, eating appropriate foods that your body can digest properly is what is going to help you obtain the majority of your health and weight loss goals. Exercise maybe plays a part, possibly, but not mostly.

I know that sentence sounds weak….I get into the explanation much more in week 2 of my *Coach Me Course*. It is basically an entire week of explaining how traditional exercise can actually hurt your weight loss efforts, while the right types of exercises will excel your program with minimal effort. Yes, this information is as life changing as it sounds! Especially if you are the chronic over-exerciser I used to be.

The next three blogs are going to touch on some of this healing foods I mention above, as well as other tricks I have used to heal myself: the good, the bad and the oh-my-lord-you-are-not-sticking-that-up-my-butt!

# *Whatchu Missing Willis?*

Since starting your new diet, have you noticed your hair falling out? No, not you pulling it out because your toddler just asked to go outside for the fifteenth time since waking up twenty minutes ago, but actually falling out?

Ask any woman who has recently given birth about losing hair by the handfuls. It happens because of all of those changing hormones. It's not bad enough that you just pushed out this screaming ball of goo, followed by the most painful poop one should never have to endure, but now your hair is clinging to every part of your body except your head. Hormones.

Guess what happens when you drastically change your diet. That's right, hormones! The good news when you eat for your hormones is you are no longer chained to calorie counting or endless cardio sessions. The bad news, sometimes your hair falls out.

There is a solution to prevent premature balding on your new diet. You can have your fats and eat them too! (Does that saying befuddle anyone else? Of course if you have cake, or fats, you want to eat them).

Ok. Eat your fats, not the cake, and then add in some collagen protein. After a few weeks of an ounce of collagen per day, poof! Your hair will be luxurious and it will stay on your head where it belongs. Not in the drain. Not hanging all over your clothes. Not in your toddler's mouth.

I know what you're thinking: collagen has a lot of protein - what about gluconeogenesis? Wait, that wasn't the first thought that crossed your mind? You must be new here. If you are worried about gluconeogenesis, just chill out on all of that for a minute. It actually occurs much less than the keto experts lead you to believe. I too was worried about this and dropped collagen from my diet for awhile. Wanna know what happened? My hair fell out. I mean, are you even paying attention?

I noticed something else happen as well.

I have a three year old that is an extremely picky eater. When I say extreme, I mean the kid won't even eat an ice cream cone. He licks the ice cream with the very tip of his tongue and then whips the cone to the ground while gagging like we just forced castor oil down his throat. He also does not eat meat. *He will eat _peanut butter fat bombs_ though. Score!*

Knowing what I know about health, he needed to get some more high quality protein into his diet. I started putting a scoop of collagen protein into his low sugar juice one to two times per day. Silly boy, he even asks for it because I told him it is sugar. The truths we parents stretch.

## *Healthy Immune System: Collagen For the Win!*

This past winter I noticed everyone in the house catching colds more than normal. Everyone except the toddler. The rest of his diet is not great. I do the best I can with what I have to work with, but there is only so much an at-the-end-of-her-rope-why-won't-you-just-eat-something-for-the-love-of-all-things-Mickey-Mouse mom can do. After waking up with one too many scratchy throats, it came to me. The collagen! He was the only one in the house still taking collagen consistently. My husband and I were so paranoid about that long G word that we immediately eliminated this healing protein from our diets. Collagen also has a long list of other health benefits beyond keeping your follicles securely attached. It is a protein our body *NEEDS* to function properly. This is one of the reasons bone broth is all the rage – collagen!

I added collagen back into my diet recently. Hello healthy immune system. I missed you. Please don't ever leave me again. What I do not miss is pulling out 3 fistfuls of brown and gray strands every time I gather my hair into a ponytail. My husband does not miss cleaning the shower drain daily and my toddler does not miss the mommy strings that end up in his mouth.

If you are still worried about gluconeogenesis, experiment with yourself. Add it to your diet and test your ketones later that day. Still in ketosis? See, it wasn't a problem. If by some small chance it does kick you out of ketosis, maybe drop those pork rinds or cheese sticks. Your health is well worth this small sacrifice. Maybe try not to take your collagen with a heavy protein meal and add some fat with your collagen dose to slow the absorption down.

If you have no clue what gluconeogenesis is, maybe try Google. Then run, don't walk, to your computer and order collagen right now. I mean, why are you still reading this? Your collagen should be in the process of being packed up by Thrive Market right now, but instead you're still reading.

There are a lot of articles out there stating all of the health benefits of a high quality collagen. Today Google will be your friend. The kind of collagen I buy is Great Lakes collagen in the green can. Green is important. The green can dissolves in hot and cold water, so you can mix it in with anything that has some flavor. I would not recommend adding it to plain water. I mean, if you have a strong stomach and no sense of smell, it's all you. I find it dissolves best if you add half of your chosen liquid to your glass, scoop in collagen and then pour the remaining liquid. Stir and let it sit for a minute or two to fully dissolve.

I currently mix collagen in with Jigsaw Electrolyte Supreme (found on Amazon, because I'm a mom and packing up two kids to shop isn't my idea of a fun day). Electrolytes + collagen + a fat bomb or two. Health perfection!

If you stopped reading this blog to order your collagen from <u>Thrive Market</u> and it just arrived at your door but you have no clue what to do with it, I have some suggestions:

- As stated above, add it to your favorite electrolyte mix. Two for one!
- Dissolve a tablespoon into your morning coffee, and then another into your afternoon coffee.
- If you adore chocolate as much as I do and do not live in the summer hades that is Arizona, make a <u>keto hot chocolate</u> and stir some in.
- Whip up some tasty <u>Chocolate Protein Cupcakes</u>. I have these listed under dessert, but I definitely eat them for breakfast.

Please do not add collagen to juice that is not for your toddler, because if you are drinking liquid sugar in the form of juice, what the heck are you doing reading a health blog anyway?!?!

# About That Noxema Girl...

## Let's Talk Girl Talk

Let me bring you back to 1990 for a minute. Aqua-netted hair as high as the heavens was all the rage, Madonna was busy teaching the world to vogue and I discovered the game Girl Talk – A Game of Truth or Dare. My ten year old self felt so cool playing such a grown up game with all of my ten year old girlfriends. I seriously lived for sleepovers where we got to bust this game open and act like the teenage girls we voraciously studied in the *Sweet Valley High* book series.

The part of that game I absolutely despised was when you did not take the genius dare another preteen girl suggested, you had to wear a zit sticker on your face. At age ten my hormones weren't quite crazy yet and my skin was still soft, hydrated and smooth. Still, the embarrassment I felt putting a zit sticker on my face was awful. I could never imagine the horror a real life zit would bring. No thank you, I will skip that phase of life.

That was the plan anyway. Then I became a teenager and the acne hit hard. It was far more embarrassing than the Girl Talk game ever lead me to believe. This was right around the time I started wearing makeup, so I was able to cover up my horrid skin a little, but the truth was still visible beneath my CoverGirl two shades too dark for me foundation.

A lot of people pin acne as a teenager's problem. Hormones are shifting, junk food is plentiful and caked on makeup is applied at the start of every single high school class. My issues with acne lasted well into my early 30's, as is the case with many women these days. I am not talking a zit or two appearing on my chin as the time of the month known as Shark Week approaches. And for those of you who think Shark Week is just a week long series on the Discovery Channel as I did, look it up on Urban Dictionary. For the longest time I couldn't figure out why so many women posted about craving junky carbs while watching sharks swim the waters on TV.

## Twenty Years of "Solutions"

I was not like a lot of my friends who complained of a small pimple or two every month. I had huge, pus filled cystic acne spots all over my self-conscious face. For twenty years I did everything I could to stop this problem in its tracks. I was a regular at the dermatologist's office and was pretty much paying to be a product tester for every single over counter solution on the market.

I tried creams, lotions, alcohol based wipes and expensive mineral makeup. I dutifully washed my face in the morning, before bed and sometimes in the middle of the day. I bought so much Proactiv that I am surprised Rodan & Fields did not ask me to star in their commercials.

On second thought, I would not have made a great after picture. Before – yes! I was their perfect before model. *Maybe* if they cast me in the commercial after the first month, that would have worked, but after the first month of applications the Proactiv was no longer my savior. You think I would have learned that lesson after buying it year after year, hoping this time would be different.

As if that list is not extensive enough, I opted for the mac daddy of all acne solutions not once, but twice. I signed on the dotted line for Accutane. After years of over the counter solutions and medical prescriptions failed me, I went to my trusted dermatologist for the end-my-pizza-face-forever solution. If you never tried Accutane, this may not sound like a big deal to you. At the time, I thought it was just a pill I popped twice per day. I'm not sure what would leave me to believe this, as it was harder to obtain an Accutane prescription than to get into Studio 54 if you weren't over the top flamboyant or a celebrity of some sort. Now I am horrified at what this innocent looking pill may have done to my body.

I suppose it is not all that innocent looking. On every single pill you take there is an image of a pregnant woman with a big red X over it. This pill was so strong that pregnant women were not even supposed to look at it. I was sworn to taking birth control while on it, and I had to sign a waiver that I would have an abortion if I did get pregnant. Thankfully I had no pregnancy plans, but how awful that is the procedure just to clear up acne. This does not even get into the horrible side effects of this wonder drug.

My skin was never so dry in my entire life. How am I supposed to use my two shades too dark CoverGirl with peeling skin covering my face? The moistness on my lips completely went away. I looked like a bit of a clown with peeling skin around my entire mouth for months. There was not enough Carmex in the world to keep my lips soft. My nose was so dry that it felt like I was being stabbed in the nostrils with sewing needles and I don't think I could even cry actual tears of pain from my dehydrated eyes.

Accutane is also associated with feeling dizzy, nervous, drowsy, back pain and joint pain. None of these symptoms were foreign to my mid-twenty something self, and Accutane exacerbated every single one! Wonder drugs of the twenty first century.

I willingly took this horrid medical solution twice. The long lasting miracle effects from this, a drug that was to cure my acne woes forever, lasted less than a year both times I endured the medication and its side effects. After a year I was back to buying the entire acne aisle at Walgreens.

For twenty years I scoured every book for the cure and never, and I mean never, left the house without a ton of caked on makeup to cover my scarlet letter. As with many things in life, if only I had known then what I know now. As in, those medications I was taking to clear up my acne were actually doing far more damage than they were ever helping. The over the counter creams, even the really pricey ones, could never fix a problem that was a result of internal issues I needed to deal with in order to rid myself of cystic acne forever.

## *Clearing Things Up:*

In early 2014 I came across the book *Kick Your Fat in the Nuts*. As mentioned before, I attempted everything in my arsenal to take off more than 100 pounds that would not budge via any other method. I consistently recycled the same three to four pounds. I decided to throw a Hail Mary and attempt the methods in this book.

I studied nutrition for the prior twenty plus years, yet a lot of the information in this book was all new to me. Nothing I previously studied was helping me in my time of desperate need, so out with the old and in with the might as well give this a try and then find something else when this doesn't work.

Except this time, this really worked! As in, I was able to lose and easily keep off over 145 pounds worked. As in, I hit my weight loss goal for the first time in my life worked, and then I lowered the goal and got there too. Not only that, but in the process I was able to finally correct so many symptoms I dealt with for more than two decades. While you can read about all of the ailments I improved in other blogs, this blog was sent here to save the day for all of the acne sufferers of the world!

The information I learned from the *Kick Your Fat in the Nuts* book, and had reinforced with their *Kick it Naturally* podcast and 12 Week Fat Loss Course, helped me figure out what twenty years of doctor's advice, over the counter solutions and clear skin infomercials could not. I was able to correct malfunctions in my body that were causing the cystic acne to continuously take up residence on my face. This improved my situation once and for all.

I found out years of prescription medications and processed foods that I was using to improve my health were actually the very things destroying my health and causing painful acne. These included years of Lean Cuisines, "healthy" whole grain products, birth control and the medical prescriptions given to me to clear up my skin. All of these products were contributing to making my bile sludgy and sticky, which prevented me from digesting food appropriately.

Years of low fat diets also contributed to this, as once your remove necessary healthy fats from your diet, your body forgets how to process these. I did everything the experts told me to do for perfect health, only to continuously fall down a rabbit hole of worsening symptoms and plus size pants.

As you can imagine, this problem did not correct itself overnight. I started with the supplement regimen outlined in book and <u>12 Week Fat Loss Course</u>. Following this routine was my Hail Mary I prayed would work. You do not need to throw up a Hail Mary – you get to learn firsthand from all of my spectacular results.

## *Let's Get Personal:*

The supplement regimen consisted of three supplements: Beet Flow, Beatine HCL and Digestizyme. While the Beatine HCL and Digestizyme are mini health miracles in their own rights, Beet Flow is the star of my healthy skin glow.

Beet Flow consists of highly concentrated beet greens. And yes, you can get the same effects of Beet Flow if you consume beet greens in your diet, however, you will need to consume one million buckets. OK, maybe not one million and maybe I watched *Austin Powers* one million times, but beet greens would be pretty much the only thing you eat every day just to get the same effect. Maybe take the pills and try to eat something more delicious.

I took Beet Flow as suggested in the book and things did start to improve. Weight was coming off, I was no longer nauseous at the sight of a steak and I began pooping everyday! I know, probably way more information than you want to know about me. Hold on tight because this blog is about to get waaaaaayyyyy more personal. This is for your benefit. My skin is clear, I have my benefit - now let's work on you.

While I followed all of the steps in the book, my skin was still a zit-filled mess. Everything else was going according to plan, so I reached out to the Kick Your Fat Support Group to get more answers. The helpful coaches told me to try Xeneplex and then follow it up the next day with a Beet Flow Flush.

I went to Natural Reference to find out what this Xeneplex was. $89 for only ten pills is what this Xeneplex was. WOAH! That seemed pricey, especially considering all of the supplements I recently added to my regimen. Then I thought about the countless acne products I tried over the course of my life and would continue to need if I never fixed the root of my problem. Suddenly a one time charge of $89 seemed like a steal. Cool. Ship me the Xeneplex! Ship me *all* the Xeneplex! (as long as it is just the one box for $89; stuff ain't cheap).

I received Xeneplex and read the instructions. I did notice it is a coffee suppository product when I ordered it. The support group told me it is used to help extra sludgy bile get moving, but I did not really take into account by what means. I found out you take the Beet Flow to attack sticky bile from one angle (taken by mouth), while Xeneplex attacks the problem from a completely different angle (taken by butt).

Yes, you read that correctly. Taken by butt. Sure that's what suppository means, but I never had to take anything like that before so I didn't really take the time to think about it. So you mean to tell me I just paid $89 for only ten pills, and if that wasn't bad enough, I had to stick these pills in my butt. They did not even have the decency to buy me a glass of wine first.

The thought of sticking a pill into my butt made me break out into cold sweats. I was cut in half a year prior, and for some reason a c-section birth seemed like child's play compared to this step. I also researched before I attempted this and read I had to hold this in for at least fifteen minutes. I didn't even understand what that all meant. This was all strange and new to me, however, I paid $89 and I was sick of pus mountains all over my face, so I took the long, lonely walk to the bathroom, I grabbed some Vasoline and I took that pill by butt.

Truth be told, I stressed for nothing. A little bit of oil came out, but other than that, life went on and I went from worrying about my own butt back to wiping my baby's butt. I followed up the next day by adding a Beet Flow flush. My bile was incredibly stubborn, so I had to follow this procedure a few times before I received the results I wanted. I already paid for the pills, so it wasn't a big deal. It's not like I planned on lending my leftover butt pills to my friends.

This fairytale come to life was about three years ago. Guess which girl still has perfect skin. If you guessed the girls in the Proactiv commercials, probably not. If you guessed me, you are paying attention! No more wasted money on creams, lotions, over the counter solutions or medical prescriptions. Heck, I barely wash my face anymore unless I am taking off makeup. (I'm a busy mom; don't judge me).

# *Learn Your Truth:*

Many people do notice their skin clears up when they start a ketogenic diet and they never had to take all of these steps. I believe this is because they are ridding themselves of processed junk food and "healthy" whole grains. This will help their bile flow more freely. Others will actually notice their skin gets worse. This also makes sense because you are adding a lot of fat to your diet, and if your bile is not flowing correctly those fats will become toxic to you. Your body may try to get rid of the toxins through the skin. This can result in acne and itchy skin.

While these steps may not be necessary for everyone, just know there is help out there for those of us who cannot get rid of acne any other way. Clear skin is one of the best indicators of good health. If your skin is not as glowing and radiant as you see in after pictures of the infomercials, definitely learn more about how to improve your digestion here. You could change your health forever for only fifty cents.

While this blog talks about obtaining the benefits of better bile flow for clearer skin, also know there are plenty of other reasons you want good bile flow. These include processing fats correctly to help stabilize blood sugar and break your reliance on carbohydrates for energy and helping a body that is dealing with diarrhea, constipation, nausea, gas, itchy skin, bloating or elevated cholesterol.

I am not some genius who had an epiphany and suddenly all of this information came to me. I learned about how to improve this health problem, along with countless others, in the 12 Week Online Fat Loss Course that I won't stop talking about. I only mention it so much because I care about you and your health. Three years ago I set out on a mission to lose fat, while I gained knowledge that will help me and my family maintain optimal health for life.

If you click through my link, the course is also only $89. If I could have learned the information taught in this course twenty years ago, I think I would have bought all the courses! To me, my health is that valuable.

Beet Flow and Xeneplex can be found at Natural Reference. Please use my practitioner code: nissahelpsme at checkout and email me for additional information.

Now who is up for a round of Girl Talk?

# My Dear Stevia Letter

I have something to tell you and I am warning you that you are not going to like it. This is something I learned last summer and probably read about long before that, but I stuck my fingers in my ears while screaming "la, la, la – 1-2-3, not it!" Ok, so I did not literally scream out loud. My four year old who jumps, kicks and shrieks for a living would have looked at me like I was nuts, but you get the idea. I read it, I checked my results in the mirror and I smugly said to myself, "Nope, nope, nope."

Part of my lack of willingness to accept this truth was due to my outstanding results. The other part was I just didn't want to accept it. I had already given up so much to live this low-carb, high-fat lifestyle. While all of the changes have been so beneficial and I have had amazing results for the first time in my life, mentally I did not want to give up one more thing, even if giving it up would make me feel even better. Especially one more thing that I used daily and did not seem to interfere with my goal in anyway. Still, I kept hearing the same advice over and over. Advice I denied over and over.

## Parting Is Such Sweet Sorrow:

After further research and self experimentation, I have finally come to the depressing realization that stevia is not my friend. Never has been, never will be.

I say depressing because the thought of a fat bomb never again touching my lips is almost unbearable. (This is that dramatic flair I mentioned in my last blog). Fat bombs have become essential in my life. I pop a few in for breakfast; have some as a snack; eat a few more as an after dinner mint. I am not me if I am not reaching for a fat bomb at any given point during the day. I'm the same girl that keeps trying to make #fatbombfriday a thing. Oh stevia, how have you done me so wrong?!?! (Again with the drama).

But you see, constantly reaching for a fat bomb throughout the day should have been my first clue that stevia really was causing problems in my high-fat, low-carb diet. I still firmly believe that many people can benefit from the healthy fats that make up most fat bomb recipes, but when you are constantly reaching for them, fat is not the only thing adding up. Most fat bombs also contain some carbs and protein. While one or two fat bombs in a day will not make much of a dent for most people, the carbs and protein can really add up when you start popping fat bomb after fat bomb all day long.

Not only were the carbs from fat bombs starting to add up for me, but so were the carb cravings. I found myself sneaking bites of food from my kids plates here and there. Ever since I took the time to improve my <u>digestion</u>, I rarely had cravings for my former favorites like fries or chips. All of the sudden it was becoming harder to control myself when faced with these options. I even sometimes secretly tasted an Annie's Organic Bunny Fruit Snack. Gasp! The shock and horror of it all!

Between the fat bombs and occasional bunnies inexplicably hopping into my mouth, the scale started changing its mind. At the time I thought maybe the scale was on an upward trajectory because of some unwelcome stress in my life. I thought once that situation calmed itself, life would get back to normal and I could resume occasionally peeling my off my momiform of yoga pants every now and then to slip into a pair of jeans without fear. Also, let's face it – the holiday season, complete with traveling with small kids, is no help for anyone hoping to keep their muffin top minimized.

## *Not So Sweet After All:*

I have not been a fan of most artificial sweeteners for some time. Once upon a time I had an addiction to Low Carb Monster drinks and occasionally sipped on Diet Coke; if you consider everyday as occasional use. Clearly in denial, I told myself that Diet Coke was an only every once in a while habit. The more I dug into other people's research, the more I learned these sweeteners were having a big impact on my health, while also making sustainable weight loss much more difficult. I started reducing my use of artificially flavored drinks until I just did not need them any longer. If I attempt to drink a diet pop now (shout out Midwesterners), it actually burns going down. An esophagus lit ablaze is an excellent reason to stay far away from the fizzy stuff.

While giving up the sodas, the carbs and the chemicals, I wanted something in my life to make me feel normal. A lot of my favorite low-carb experts said *some* artificial sweeteners are perfectly fine for everyday use. I trusted their word and I used these sweeteners daily. As I dug more into research, I settled on liquid stevia as my sweetener of choice. The powdered stuff had additives I didn't want and I had bad personal experiences with Swerve. Most other artificial sweeteners have been shown to raise blood sugar, although I am sure you can find studies that also show the opposite. Some studies have sponsors. Sometimes nefarious sponsors who skew the results. Whether or not this was the case, I found it best to steer clear.

The negative Nancies persisted and continued to bash my precious savior liquid stevia. (Does anyone else instantly picture Jeffrey Dean Morgan swinging a barbed wire baseball bat when you hear the word savior these days? Yes I watch The Real Housewives and The Walking Dead. I'm diverse like that).

In any case, I stopped using stevia while fasting long ago because I did notice a rise in hunger soon after using stevia in coffee. A rise in hunger while fasting most likely means an insulin spike. An insulin spike with no food coming in immediately welcomes your body into fat storing mode. Fat storing mode is not a welcome guest in my household.

# But We Were On A Break!

In November I made the decision to cut back stevia a little to see how I would do. I started to add less stevia to the fat bomb recipes I was making. To be honest, I didn't really notice a big difference in taste, even when cutting the amount used to half or even a fourth. My husband actually preferred the new recipes with less sweeteners.

Lets fast forward to January, because December was just a big old holiday mess of not sticking to anything much of the time, thanks in part to neighbors who bring trays of cookies and treats to make us fat for the holidays.

Does the *Eating Fat is the New Skinny* logo on my SUV mean nothing to them? I may need a *Beware of Carbs* sign on my door. Delivery men have laughed out loud at my *Beware of Dog* sign, you know, since my dog is full grown and weighs seven pounds. Not to mention she runs under my feet in the presence of strangers. A *Beware of Carbs* sign will probably be much more effective at keeping unwanted strangers out. I don't imagine many masked robbers restrict their carbs, much less think they will find anything of value in a home warning them of the dangers of sugar and bread!

Completely unrelated tangents aside, in January I was a little worried about how I was going to get back on track. I decided getting back to an intermittent fasting routine would be the best thing to help Nissa get her groove back. (Shout out Angela Bassett movie I have never watched, yet love to reference). Damn those unrelated tangents. You would think I would just go back and edit them out.

# It's Like I Never Even Knew You:

While looking for inspiration on getting back to an intermittent fasting routine, I came across a book that absolutely forbid artificial sweeteners during the fasting window. Point noted, already followed. But this author also talked about not using artificial sweeteners while eating. She actually even sometimes drinks Coke – as in the real stuff. I'm talking actual liquid sugar, the most insulin spiking substance in the land. She wrote while she sometimes drinks Coke, she no longer uses artificial sweeteners in any capacity.

But come on, surely she did not mean stevia. Multiple studies have told me stevia is fine. All of my favorite health experts told me stevia is great. Not a single one would recommend Coke in place of Zevia. Who was this crazy loon and how did she even get a book deal?

To make matters worse, as I read further I found out she did in fact mean stevia. She said while she was able to make it to her goal weight with the use of stevia, she was struggling with dreaded weight regain. While I do not recall writing this diet book, I felt like I could have. Minus the Coke part, because Coke and I will never be on a first name basis like that.

Backing up to the mean name calling part – I never really considered her a crazy loon. I think I was just mad that what she was saying made sense and that meant I had to say goodbye to my beloved. I actually adored the fact that her long diet history mirrored mine and she finally found food freedom after decades of diet disasters. Sounds all too familiar. I continued to read her very well researched  book and paid close attention.

## *It's Not You, It's Me. On Second Thought, It's Totally You:*

Most experts say stevia is ok because it does not spike blood glucose. Perhaps that is true. This author cites the reason to give up stevia is it has been shown to spike insulin. Holy fat bomb, now she is speaking my language. Less drastic insulin spikes lead to less weight gain and less cravings. The real kicker is she found this information in the exact book I found it in last summer. The one where I stuck my fingers in my ears before popping another stevia filled fat bomb. There the information was dangling in front of my face all along and I was too smug to listen.

This time around I paid more attention. I immediately stopped adding stevia to all of the recipes I made. I even went so far as to throw a few bags of fat bombs away. I know, blasphemy! Even more shock and horror! But if there was a chance they were working against me, I wanted to test and find out for myself. No more trusting random studies or even my favorite experts who say they are fine. The only way to know if these sweeteners were only sweet talking me to get into my pants was to test for myself. And by get into my pants, I mean making them tighter. Let it be known I am not attempting to add stevia to the #metoo movement. That would be weird. And unfair.

Now that I have spent an entire blog bashing what may be your last low-carb hope, I bet you are wondering about the results I experienced. Or you hate me. It could go either way at this point.

The good news is, I no longer see this as a depressing realization. Eliminating all artificial sweeteners from my diet this past month has been absolutely life changing for me. It has helped so much with appetite correction that I no longer am constantly reaching for more fat bombs throughout the day. In fact, there are days I do not even eat fat bombs because I am just not hungry. My body is doing an awesome job of craving real, whole foods that will help it function most optimally now that it is not dealing with constant artificially sweetened insulin spikes throughout the day.

In case you are wondering how I am still eating fat bombs but not stevia, well that's easy. I just don't add sweeteners to the recipes. In some cases it is easy to just leave them out completely, like with these <u>Caramel Apple Fat Bombs</u>. In other recipes I have switched to something with just a little sweetness like 88% dark chocolate, like with these <u>Unsweetened Peanut Butter Fat Bombs</u>. Once you give your body and taste buds ample time to adjust, these fat bombs are sweet enough to be considered a treat.

I am sure the keto police are suited up and ready to berate me for the little bit of sugar hiding out in the dark chocolate. Many are more than happy to spike insulin all day long with artificial sweeteners, but all holy hell will break loose at the mere mention of a natural added sugar to a recipe. Fingers will be pointed and recipes will be banned.

Everybody just calm down for a minute. By the time I melt down the two or so ounces over 24 fat bombs, there is more than enough taste with very little sugar per bomb. Plus I have come to the ultimate realization that my body knows how to process that sugar. My body is providing just enough insulin to process the real food source instead of being confused by sugar it thinks is coming, but never actually arrives.

The other good news – I went to a delicious steak dinner last week and buttoned my jeans with no unsightly muffin top hangover. That did not happen two weeks ago. Yet another stevia-free victory – I brought home my beloved bunless Bacon Bacon Burger from The Cheesecake Factory and did not steal even one of my son's fries on the drive home. Previously I was all, "Huh, I don't know what happened to the fries. I guess they don't fill those bags the way they used to. Nope, don't know anything about the salt all over my face."

# *IN CONCLUSION:*

Ha. Look at me ending this blog like I am all sciencey.

While I am not sciencey in the least, as proven by my choice of the word sciencey, I am a bona fide health geek. Not so much of a geek that I go back and read every interesting study I come across, but that's mostly because ain't nobody got time for that. Once a subject interests me, as "natural" artificial sweeteners currently does, I tend to read as much as I can as quickly as I can.

While reading up on how stevia affects insulin levels, I came across some articles that show not only can stevia raise insulin levels, but it can also increase abdominal fat, cravings and man boobs.

That being said, there is also a plethora of articles out there touting the health benefits of stevia. While it is too early for me to notice any other positive health benefits beyond just feeling more in control, some of the articles I found are enough to make me quit the artificially sweet stuff for good. Only the future knows if I will finally be able to rid myself of a chunk of stubborn belly fat that previously promised to always be mine.

Am I telling you to never use artificial sweeteners in your diet? Nope, nope, nope. The truth is I am so excited about the results I have had thus far with removing all artificial sweeteners from my diet that I wanted to share my results with anyone else who may be questioning stevia . In fact, the only person I will tell not to use artificial sweeteners is myself because I simply feel better throughout the day without them. I realize that may not be the case for everyone reading this blog. Well, and also my husband, because you know, man boobs.

# Thank you!

Thank you so much for sticking with me through my health journey via these blogs I penned over the course of the past year. For even more witty insight on health topics, visit my website www.eatingfatisthenewskinny.com. I have plenty more health musings, life lessons and entertaining articles for your viewing pleasure.

AND I HAVE CHOCOLATE! I had to yell that because chocolate is important. My weight loss transformation was recently showcased on channel 12 Phoenix News as the featured news story for the evening. The news teaser that led into the 10 pm news was a close up of me telling all of Phoenix, which is the 11th leading news market in the nation, "Half of my diet consists of dark chocolate."

It's funny, but it's true! I eat a lot of delicious dark chocolate combined with healthy fats. In order to keep my fats high on my low-carb, high-fat diet, I eat a lot of chocolate fat bombs. De-lish! If you want to see me in all of my chocolate fat bomb glory, click here.

Find even more of my delicious recipes in *The Lazy Keto Gourmet*. This book contains the real meals I ate to lose more than 100 pounds and the meals I still eat to maintain. I also include tips throughout the book on how to best use these meals and treats for maximum fat burning.

If you want even more of these tips that saved me from a life of desperation and fat girl clothes, enroll in my *Coach Me Course: Escape Diet Mentality and End Yo-Yo Diets Forever*. There is waaaaaayyyyyy more to this fabulous lifestyle than move more, eat less...especially since that's not really even a real thing!

People can scream, "Keto and IF!" at you all day long - but do you even know what in the bologna sandwiches they are talking about? And if you are still eating bologna sandwiches, YOU NEED MY COURSE IN YOUR LIFE NOW!

If you want to take your health progress to the next level, sign up for my _Teach Me Course_. This is the combo package of my six week motivational course combined with the 12 Week Online Fat Loss Course that changed my life forever! You will not find any greater health knowledge out there...especially in a discounted combo deal!

# More About Nissa Graun:

I followed mainstream diet advice for more than twenty five years. I was constantly sick, tired and miserable for the majority of those two plus decades. Sometimes I lost weight, but it was always a difficult process and the weight was routinely gained back within a year, plus more. The chronic illness always remained a constant.

After hitting an all time high weight of 245 pounds after the birth of my first child, I felt completely helpless. All of my previous methods of weight loss were absolutely useless. I was fat, sick, and miserable while still wearing maternity clothes many months after the birth of my first son.

I came across a book and course that changed my life. I learned how to use natural supplements and nutrition to not only take off the weight, but also improve all of the health issues that had been plaguing me longer than I can remember. I set out with intentions of dropping weight that was not budging via any other method, while unintentionally correcting many health problems that afflicted me for decades. These include chronic heartburn, cystic acne, frequent migraines and headaches, frequent sinus infections, constant drippy nose, itchy skin, insomnia, nausea, frequent anxiety, constipation, occasional depression, hypoglycemia, diabetic level blood sugars and constant junk food cravings, just to name a few.

Four years later I am thriving. Keeping the weight off has been a piece of cake. Oh, and I no longer want to eat cake. My weight is now at my lowest point and easily maintained. Now that my digestion is healed and I know the foods that keep me satisfied, living life no longer feels like work. For the first time in my life the constant food noise is gone and I am left with food freedom.

While I have always been passionate about health, I finally know what true health feels like. My passion is to help others achieve their optimal health as well through my blogs, recipes and personal health coaching.

Join my Facebook group    Follow me on Instagram    Follow Me on Facebook

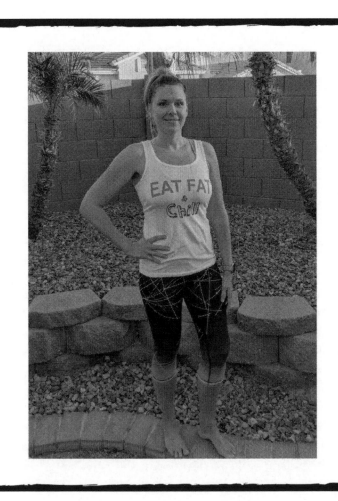

Made in the USA
Middletown, DE
15 April 2019